WORKBOOK

MATERNAL NEWBORN NURSING

FOURTH EDITION

Marcia L. London, RNC, MSN, NNP
Associate Professor and
Director of Neonatal Nurse Practitioner Program
Beth-El College of Nursing
Colorado Springs, Colorado

Patricia W. Ladewig, PhD, RNC, NP
Professor and Dean
School for Health Professions
Regis University
Denver, Colorado

Sally B. Olds, RNC, MS
Associate Professor
Beth-El College of Nursing
Colorado Springs, Colorado

ADDISON-WESLEY NURSING
A Division of The Benjamin/Cummings Publishing Company, Inc.
Redwood City, California • Menlo Park, California
Reading, Massachusetts • New York • Don Mills, Ontario
Wokingham, U.K. • Amsterdam • Bonn • Sydney
Singapore • Tokyo • Madrid • San Juan

Sponsoring Editor   Patti Cleary
Production Coordinator   Cathy Lewis
Cover Quilt   "The Tide" by Miwako Kimura
Cover Designer   Yvo Riezebos
Copyeditor   Mary Prescott
Proofreader   Holly McLean-Aldis
Composition   ExecuStaff

Credits: Chapter opening photographs for Chapters 1, 2, 3, 5, 6, 8-15 by Elizabeth Elkin. Chapter opening photographs 4 and 7 by Amy Snyder.

We dedicate this book to our families—with love.
David, Craig, and Matthew London
Tim, Ryan, and Erik Ladewig
Joe, Scott, and Allison Olds

ISBN   0-8053-5584-7
 5 6 7 8 9 10-CRS-97 96 95 94

ADDISON-WESLEY NURSING
A Division of The Benjamin/Cummings Publishing Company, Inc.
Redwood City, California • Menlo Park, California
Reading, Massachusetts • New York • Don Mills, Ontario
Wokingham, U.K. • Amsterdam • Bonn • Sydney
Singapore • Tokyo • Madrid • San Juan

Contents

Preface

Maternal-newborn nurses are responsible for a complex, highly specialized body of knowledge related to the needs of the child-bearing family, whether normal or at-risk. In recent years, that knowledge has expanded rapidly, as have the technology and complex ethical issues surrounding pregnancy and birth.

Nursing programs must deal with this explosion of knowledge and with the complex bioethical issues. The *Maternal-Newborn Nursing Workbook* can assist in that effort by providing a concise, up-to-date review of essential theoretical content, emphasizing application of the nursing process and critical thinking in clinical maternity settings.

The subject areas included in this workbook were chosen to assist students in learning the most essential content of maternal-newborn nursing. In addition, selected women's health issues are explored.

All major maternity texts include content related to the human reproductive system and to the antepartal, intrapartal, postpartal, and neonatal periods, although their sequences may vary. This workbook can be used with most of the major maternity nursing texts, no matter what their organization. It is specifically designed to be used with Olds-London-Ladewig, *Maternal-Newborn Nursing: A Family-Centered Approach*, 4th edition and the subjects follow the same sequences as in the textbook. The workbook is appropriate for all types of nursing programs—baccalaureate, associate degree and diploma. Nurses involved in refresher courses or just entering this specialty area will also find it helpful. Practicing nurses may find it helpful, too, especially in assessment and critical clinical decision-making.

Chapter 1 introduces pertinent maternal-child nursing concepts and reviews examples of relevant statistical data. It includes a brief overview of selected theories related to the family as well as societal issues, such as family violence, that affect the childbearing woman.

Chapters 2 and 3 review anatomy and physiology of human reproduction, focusing on the physiological and psychological experience of being a woman throughout the life span.

Chapter 5 explores the physiologic and psychologic adaptations occurring in pregnancy. Chapter 6 focuses on assessment and care of the normal antepartal family, including maternal nutrition and preparation for parenthood. Chapter 7 considers the antepartal family experiencing complications. A wide range of fetal assessment

techniques, those widely used and selected newer experimental techniques, are examined in Chapter 8.

Chapters 9 through 11 consider different aspects of the intrapartal period: the physiologic and psychologic changes that occur, nursing assessment and care of the family during childbirth (including a concise review of pain relief and comfort measures) and the at-risk woman in labor and birth.

Chapter 12 includes the physiologic and psychologic responses and needs of the newborn along with appropriate nursing care measures. Chapter 13 considers the needs and care of the newborn with complications.

In a similar manner, Chapter 14 considers the normal postpartum period, and Chapter 15 is devoted to the assessment and care of the family with postpartum complications.

Features New to This Edition

This workbook emphasizes the application and synthesis of an expanding Maternal-Newborn Nursing clinical knowledge base. Since we learn best through active learning, we have provided critical thinking scenarios to further develop your critical decision making skills. An additional feature is directed toward helping the student establish priorities for nursing actions. Situations are presented and the student is asked to prioritize the actions. Action sequences have been developed for both normal and complication chapters to provide realistic clinical practice situations. Clinical data is presented and the student is guided through the decision making process for a particular situation.

Because we believe that sound clinical judgment develops from both theoretical knowledge and practical experience, most of the items in this workbook are based on clinical situations. Recognizing the rich cultural heritage of our diverse population, many of these client situations include ethnic families.

Since some students have voiced distress at the prospect of completing "care plan after care plan," we present selected portions of care plans for childbearing women and their infants. After presentation of the client situation, the student is asked to complete a portion of the care plan. For example, the nursing diagnosis may be provided and the student develops short-term goals, or evaluative outcome criteria are listed and the student identifies nursing interventions to ensure that those criteria are met.

Working with the childbearing family is an intensely rewarding interactive nursing experience. The reviewing of these clinical experiences and/or of a personal childbearing experience increases our understanding of the universal childbirth/ parenting experience. We have provided the student with opportunities in the new feature "It's Your Turn" feature to revisit and ponder those experiences.

Some of the questions are related to factual material, and students can verify their answers in any major maternity text. However, some items require synthesis and application; thus the answers may not be confirmed readily. In these instances, we have established a dialogue with the student to assist in self-assessment. If students fail to grasp certain content, they can find helpful recommendations about ways to restudy this material. Items that are reviewed in a dialogue are marked with an asterisk and addressed at the end of Part I in each chapter.

Part II of each chapter is a Self Assessment Guide. This includes a new section designed to assist the student in integrating the specialized vocabulary/abbreviations used in maternal/newborn nursing. This section also includes multiple-choice items, with answers provided. Students who have accurately completed the items in Part I should be able to answer successfully all the questions in Part II.

Clarification of Terms

Although we recognize that the men in nursing are becoming more involved in the provision of maternity care, women are still the major care providers. Therefore, whenever possible, we have avoided sexist pronouns in referring to the nurse. When this was not possible, we have used the female pronoun.

By the same token, we appreciate the fact that the individual who is most significant to the pregnant woman may be her husband, the father of the child, another family member, or simply a good friend, male or female. Thus we have provided both traditional "husband-wife" situations, and situations involving other support persons.

Acknowledgements

First, we would like to recognize the students who reviewed the previous edition of this workbook. They approached their review seriously and provided many candid comments. They identified material that they felt was unclear and added valuable suggestions that enhance this edition.

We thank the nurse educators and practicing nurses who reviewed this material and offered suggestions and comments. Their input helped us focus on the most pertinent material and offered a broader perspective.

We especially thank Patti Cleary, our editor, for her encouragement and support. To Cathy Lewis, our production coordinator, we express our appreciation for her skill in guiding the production process through to publication.

Last but not least, we thank our families. We recognize the countless ways that they continue to help us and the sacrifices that they make as we pursue this other love. Women can accomplish any goal, however, combining marriage, family, intellectual challenges and a career requires a supportive, adaptive, responsive family. Each of us is blessed with such a family. We love them.

M.L.L.
P.W.L
S.B.O.

Maternity Nursing: Changing Perspectives and Issues

1

Introduction

The broad scope of maternity nursing offers a variety of professional opportunities and greatly increases the quality of care available to childbearing families. Nurses today draw on their educational and professional expertise and also use family and statistical data in planning and providing care.

This chapter provides an introduction to the current roles of maternity nurses. It then focuses on pertinent statistical data. The latter portion of the chapter is designed to assist students in reading statistical tables and at the same time allow them to reflect briefly on the significance of the information provided in the tables.

After reviewing statistical information, the chapter introduces selected theories related to family structure, development, and functioning. This introductory content is intended to provide a base for consideration of the care required by a family during its childbearing time.

This chapter corresponds to Chapters 1, 2, and 3 in *Maternal-Newborn Nursing: A Family-Centered Approach*, 4th ed., 1992.

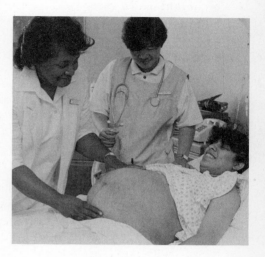

Part I Concepts, Critical Thinking, and Clinical Applications

1. Maternity nurses function in a variety of roles in providing care to childbearing families. Define each of the following roles with emphasis on educational background and scope of function:

    a. Labor and birth (clinic, postpartal, or newborn nursery) professional nurse

    b. Clinical nurse specialist

    c. Nurse practitioner

    d. Certified nurse-midwife (CNM)

2. What is meant by the term *lay midwife*?

1

3. Briefly discuss the concept of family-centered maternity care.

4. Define the following terms:

   a. Birth rate

   b. Infant death rate

   c. Neonatal mortality

   d. Perinatal mortality

   e. Maternal mortality

5. Using Table 1–1, answer the following:

   *a. The neonatal mortality rate was _____ for 1980 and _____ for 1990.

   *b. The infant death rate has changed from _____ in 1950 to _____ in 1990.

   c. Summarize the major factors you think have been important in the change of infant mortality rate from 1950 to 1990.

Table 1–1 Infant Mortality Rates by Age: United States, 1950,† 1960,† 1970,† 1980,† and 1989

Year	Under 1 year	Under 28 days	28 days–11 months
1990 (June)	9.5*	5.9*	3.5*
1989	9.7**	6.2**	3.4**
1980	12.6	8.4	4.1
1970	20.0	15.1	4.9
1960	26.0	18.7	7.3
1950	29.2	20.5	8.7

†National Center for Health Statistics: Annual summary of births, marriages, divorces, and deaths, United States, 1985. Monthly Vital Statistics Report. Vol. 34, No. 13, DHHS Pub. No. (PHS) 86–1120. Public Health Service, Hyattsville, MD. September, 19, 1986.

*National Center for Health Statistics: Births, marriages, divorces, and deaths for June 1990. Monthly Vital Statistics Report. Vol. 39, No. 6. Hyattsville, MD: Public Health Service, 1990

**National Center for Health Statistics: Annual summary of births, marriages, divorces, and deaths: United States, 1989. Monthly Vital Statistics Report. Vol. 38, No. 13. Hyattsville, MD: Public Health Service, 1990.

Table 1–2 Birth Rates by Age of Mother, Live-Birth Order, and Race of Child: United States, 1988*
[Rates are live births per 1000 women in specified age and racial group. Live-birth order refers to number of children born alive to mother.]

Live-birth order and race of child	15–44 years†	10–14 years	Total	15–19 years 15–17 years	18–19 years	20–24 years	25–29 years	30–34 years	35–39 years	40–44 years	45–49 years
All races											
Total	67.2	1.3	53.6	33.8	81.7	111.5	113.4	73.7	27.9	4.8	0.2
First child	27.6	1.3	41.0	29.1	57.9	53.1	41.2	19.1	5.7	0.8	0.0
Second child	22.0	0.0	10.3	4.2	18.9	38.0	40.8	26.4	8.4	1.1	0.0
White											
Total	63.0	0.6	43.7	25.5	69.2	102.5	111.6	72.9	26.9	4.4	0.2
First child	26.2	0.6	34.8	22.7	51.7	51.4	41.9	19.3	5.7	0.8	0.0
Second child	21.1	0.0	7.6	2.5	14.7	35.2	41.1	26.7	8.3	1.0	0.0
All other											
Total	87.5	4.0	95.3	67.6	137.4	152.3	122.3	77.8	33.4	7.0	0.4
First child	34.3	3.9	67.1	55.0	85.6	60.7	37.5	17.9	5.8	1.1	0.0
Second child	26.3	0.1	21.6	10.9	38.0	50.5	39.7	24.7	9.1	1.4	0.1
Black‡											
Total	86.6	4.8	105.9	76.6	150.5	157.5	112.8	66.0	27.5	5.6	0.3
First child	33.5	4.7	74.1	62.1	92.4	60.4	29.8	12.4	4.0	0.8	0.0
Second child	25.8	0.1	24.3	12.5	42.3	52.9	37.3	19.8	6.8	1.0	0.0

†*Rates computed by relating total births, regardless of age of mother, to women aged 15–44 years.*
‡*Included in All other.*

National Center for Health Statistics: Advance report of final natality statistics, 1988. Monthly Vital Statistics Report. Vol. 39, No. 4, Supp. Hyattsville, MD: Public Health Service, 1990. Modified from Table 3, p. 17.

6. Using Table 1–2, answer the following:

   *a. The total birth rate in 1988 for women 15–44 of all races was _____.

   b. In "all races" the highest birth rate is in the _____ to _____ age range.

   c. In the "black" category, the highest birth rate is in the age range of _____ to _____.

7. Define *family*.

8. Describe each of the following types of family configurations:

   a. Blended (stepparent) families

   b. Extended family

   c. Nuclear family

   d. Three-generation family

---

*These questions are addressed at the end of Part I.

9. Briefly discuss and compare two theoretical frameworks that may be used to evaluate families.

10. Briefly describe the various roles a nurse assumes when working with families.

11. How may an individual's perception of an adult's role or a child's role influence the care that a childbearing family receives?

Family Violence

12. Briefly discuss the social, political, psychological, and cultural factors that contribute to the incidence of spouse abuse.

13. Discuss the role of the nurse in working with an abused woman.

*14. A friend of yours says, "Women who are abused want it or else they would get out of the situation." What will you say to your friend to dispute this myth and to provide factual information?

15. Identify risk factors associated with parents who abuse their children.

16. Discuss the responsibilities of the nurse who suspects child abuse.

17. Explore the resources for abuse crisis centers in your community. Prepare a resource guide for your work with families.

---

*These questions are addressed at the end of Part I.

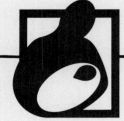

It's Your Turn

What type of family do you live in? How does it compare to the definitions given in your readings? What changes in family structure do you think have been the most important in the last ten years? What do you think the future holds for families?

_____

_____

_____

_____

_____

_____

_____

_____

_____

_____

_____

_____

_____

_____

_____

_____

Selected Answers

This section addresses the asterisked questions found in this chapter.

5. a. The neonatal mortality rate was 8.4 for 1980 and 5.9 (provisional) for 1990.

    b. The infant death rate changed from 29.2 in 1950 to 9.5 in 1990.

6. a. The total birth rate in 1988 for women 15–44 of all races was 67.2.

14. This seems a difficult myth to dispel. You may wonder why a woman stays in an abusive home. The answer is very complex, but it definitely is not because she "wants to be abused." Many women feel trapped, with no alternatives. They may have low self-esteem and therefore feel they cause the abuse and violence directed toward them. As you prepare your answer, you will need to explore your own feelings.

Part II Self-Assessment Guide

Do you know the following words?

Descriptive statistics

Inferential statistics

Can you answer the following questions?

The following multiple-choice questions will help you assess your knowledge of the content of this chapter. Select the best answer for each of the questions and then refer to the end of Part II to check your answers.

1. Which of the following would be most qualified to provide prenatal, intrapartal, postpartal, and newborn care for the low-risk childbearing woman?
    a. Acute-care clinical nurse specialist
    b. Certified nurse-midwife
    c. Lay midwife
    d. Obstetric or women's health care nurse practitioner

2. Perinatal mortality is a combination of
    a. infant death rate and neonatal mortality.
    b. fetal death rate and infant death rate.
    c. neonatal mortality and postneonatal mortality.
    d. fetal death rate and neonatal mortality.

3. You are involved in a research project designed to determine whether women seem to tolerate labor better if they are permitted to take a warm shower whenever they wish. In this case, you would be making use of the statistics you obtain to
    a. help establish a data base for different client populations.
    b. provide information about your local maternity population.
    c. evaluate the success of specific nursing interventions.
    d. determine the level of client care requirements.

4. Lisa and John and their 6-month-old son live in a duplex. Lisa's parents live in the other half of the duplex and are available any time for babysitting. In exchange, John maintains the yard and Lisa drives her mother to the doctor. What type of family configuration best describes this situation?

   a. Kin network
   b. Three-generation family
   c. Nuclear family
   d. Communal family

5. Abusive parents have many characteristics in common. Which of the following best describes their characteristics?

   a. Are well-educated, in the upper class, and have many interests
   b. Are almost always in the lower class
   c. Have many pressures they feel unable to deal with
   d. Are unskilled in crisis intervention and quickly learn new techniques once counseled

6. A nurse can help an abused woman by

   a. reporting the woman's husband and having him arrested.
   b. encouraging the woman to take her husband to a counselor.
   c. providing factual information about the cycle of abuse and suggesting resources that may be available.
   d. refusing to treat her unless she agrees to counseling.

7. When a nurse suspects child abuse she should

   a. wait until the evidence is conclusive.
   b. confront the parents and suggest counseling.
   c. remove the child from the home and keep the child until the authorities can make an appropriate placement.
   d. document the evidence and notify proper authorities immediately.

Answers

1. b   2. d   3. c   4. a   5. c   6. c   7. d

The Reproductive System and Special Reproductive Concerns

2

Introduction

Puberty is a major milestone in a young person's life. Secondary sex characteristics develop, the reproductive organs mature, and the adolescent becomes capable of procreation. This chapter reviews the female and male reproductive systems and reinforces the knowledge base from which maternity nursing care is derived.

Most couples who want children are able to have them with little difficulty. In some instances, couples may not be so fortunate and are unable to fulfill their dream of having a healthy baby because of special reproductive problems. This chapter also discusses the reproductive concern of infertility and the impact of genetics on reproduction and corresponds to Chapters 4 and 5 in *Maternal-Newborn Nursing: A Family-Centered Approach,* 4th ed.

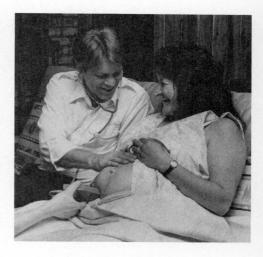

Part I Concepts, Critical Thinking, and Clinical Applications

Female Reproductive System

1. Label the structures that constitute the external female genitals on Figure 2–1.

Figure 2–1 Female external genitals, longitudinal section

2. Figure 2–2 shows the female internal reproductive organs. Identify the structures that are indicated.

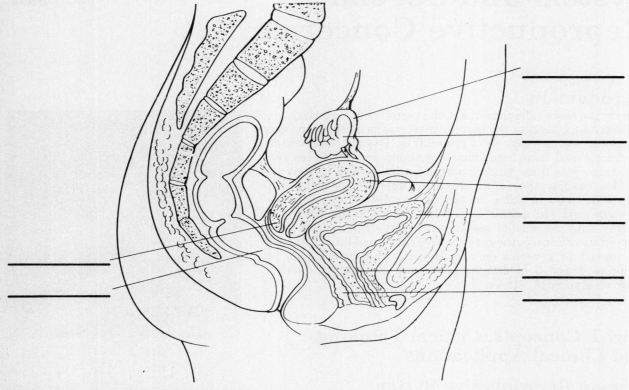

Figure 2–2 Female internal reproductive organs

3. Briefly discuss the function(s) of the vagina.

4. The acid pH of the vagina during a woman's reproductive years facilitates _____.

5. What factors alter the vagina's pH?

6. Identify three functions of the cervical mucosa.

   a.

   b.

   c.

7. Label the uterine structures indicated in Figure 2–3.

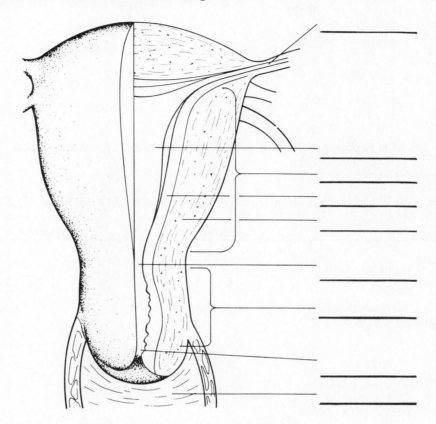

Figure 2–3   Anatomy of the uterus. (Modified from Spence AP, Mason EB: *Human Anatomy and Physiology,* 3rd ed. Menlo Park, CA: Benjamin/Cummings Publishing Co., 1987, p. 825)

8. The myometrium has three muscular layers. Identify the direction of the muscle fibers in each layer and their primary function.

Layer	Direction of Fibers	Function
Outer		
Middle		
Inner		

9. Briefly describe the function of the endometrium.

10. The two main arteries supplying blood to the uterus and fallopian tubes are the

    _____ and the _____ .

11. Identify the location and function of each of the following uterine ligaments:

Ligament	Locations	Function
Broad ligaments		
Round ligaments		
Cardinal ligaments		
Infundibulopelvic ligament		
Uterosacral ligaments		
Ovarian ligaments		

12. From what portion of the uterus do the fallopian tubes arise?

13. What are the primary functions of the fallopian tubes?

14. In relation to the fallopian tubes, what is the purpose or significance of each of the following?

   a. Fimbriae

   b. Isthmus

   c. Ampulla

   d. Peristaltic movements

   e. Nonciliated goblet cells of the mucosa

   f. Tubal cilia

15. Briefly describe the function of each of the three layers of the ovary.

   a. Tunica albuginea

   b. Cortex

   c. Medulla

16. What is (are) the primary function(s) of the ovaries?

17. Label the following pelvic bones and supporting ligaments on Figure 2–4.

Sacral body   Sacroiliac ligament
Left innominate bone   Sacrospinous ligament
Symphysis pubis   Sacrotuberous ligament
Right sacroiliac joint   Coccyx

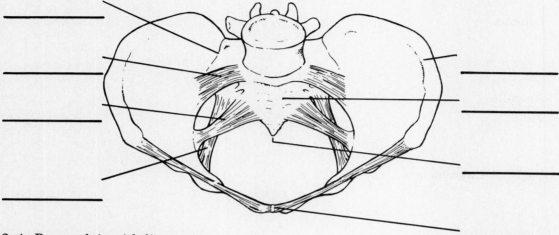

Figure 2–4 Bony pelvis with ligaments

18. Figure 2–5 focuses on the muscles of the pelvic floor. Label the following structures:

Vagina   Pudendal vessels   Pubococcygeus muscle
Bulbospongiosus muscle   Iliococcygeus muscle   External anal sphincter
Gluteus maximus muscle   Ischial tuberosity   Urogenital diaphragm
Ischiocavernosus muscle   Adductor longus muscle

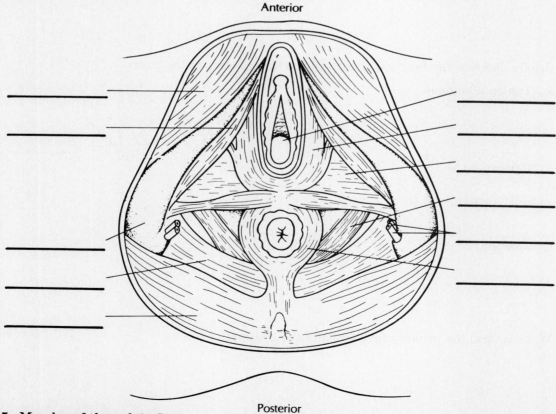

Figure 2–5 Muscles of the pelvic floor

19. The major muscle group that forms the pelvic diaphragm is the

   _____ .

20. Define each of the following terms and briefly identify its implications for childbearing:
   a. False pelvis

   b. True pelvis

   c. Pelvic inlet

   d. Pelvic outlet

21. On Figure 2–6, label the false pelvis, true pelvis, pelvic inlet, and pelvic outlet.

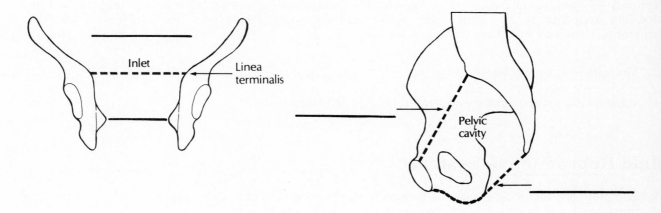

Figure 2–6 Pelvis divisions

22. Label the major structures of the breast on Figure 2–7.

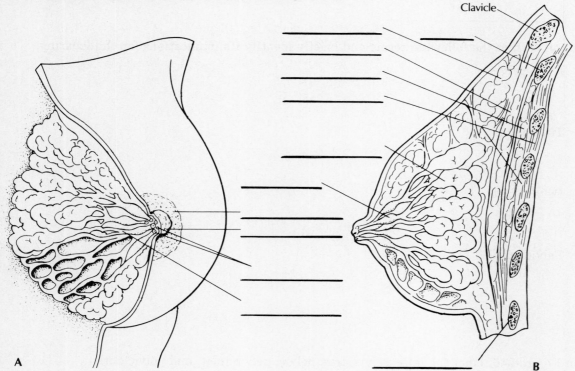

Clavicle

A

B

Figure 2–7 Anatomy of the breast. A Anterior view of partially dissected left breast. B Sagittal section. (Modified from Spence AP, Mason EB: *Human Anatomy and Physiology,* 3rd ed. Menlo Park, CA: Benjamin/Cummings Pub. Co., 1987, p. 830)

23. The nipple is composed primarily of _____ tissue.

24. What is the primary function of the tubercles of Montgomery?

Male Reproductive System

25. Complete the following sentences using the words related to the male reproductive structures and functions listed below. A word may be used more than once.

Words: Bulbourethral (Cowper's) glands, epididymides, ejaculatory duct, Leydig cells, penis, prostate gland, Sertoli cells, seminal fluid (semen), seminal vesicles, testis, testes, vas deferens.

The visible male reproductive organs include the _____ and the scrotum. The primary function of the scrotum is protection; it contains the _____ , _____ , and _____ : the male internal reproductive structures.

Each _____ produces testosterone via the _____ , which houses the seminiferous tubules and immature sperm. Maturation of sperm occurs in the _____ , the storage area for mature spermatozoa. Seminiferous tubules contain _____ cells that nourish and protect the spermatocytes. The _____ secretes fluids high in fructose and prostaglandins that nourish sperm and increase their motility. The vas deferens and the duct of a seminal vesicle unite to form a short tube called the _____ , which passes through the prostate gland and terminates in the urethra. The _____ gland secretes thin, alkaline fluid containing calcium and other substances that counteract the acidity of ductus and seminal vesicle secretions. The prostate gland secretes substances in the _____ . The _____ glands secrete viscous, alkaline fluid rich in mucoproteins, which neutralize the acid in the male urethra and the vagina.

26. The normal sperm count per ejaculation is _____ .

Puberty

27. Define *puberty*.

28. Briefly discuss the major physical changes that occur during puberty.

    a. Boys

    b. Girls

It's Your Turn

Puberty comes as a surprise to some, whereas others are well prepared. How well prepared were you for the experience? What might you do or have you done to prepare your children for puberty? What are your memories of going through puberty?

_____

_____

_____

_____

_____

_____

_____

Female Reproductive Cycle (FRC)

29. For each of the following hormones involved in ovulation and menstruation, state the source of secretion and the primary function(s).

Hormone	Source	Function
Estrogen		
Progesterone		
Follicle-stimulating hormone (FSH)		
Luteinizing hormone (LH)		
Prostaglandins (PGE and $PGF_{2\alpha}$)		

30. The female reproductive cycle is made up of two interrelated cycles that occur simultaneously: the _____ cycle and the _____ cycle.

31. Neurohumoral control of the female reproductive cycle is under the control of these three endocrine systems:

a.

b.

c.

32. Match the phase of the menstrual cycle with its related day or period of time within a 28-day cycle.

_____ Proliferative   1. Day 1–5

_____ Ischemic   2. Day 6–14

_____ Secretory   3. Day 14

_____ Menstrual   4. Day 15–26

_____ Ovulation   5. Day 27–28

33. Label the following components of the menstrual cycle on Figure 2–8 (on page **20**).

        Menstrual   Follicular

        Proliferative   Luteal

        Secretory   Estrogen

        Ischemic   Progesterone

34. Briefly decribe the changes that occur in each of the following during the various phases of the menstrual cycle.

    a. Endometrium

    b. Cervical mucosa

35. Decribe the process of ovulation and the related changes in the ovarian follicle.

36. How would you explain the process of menstruation to a group of adolescents?

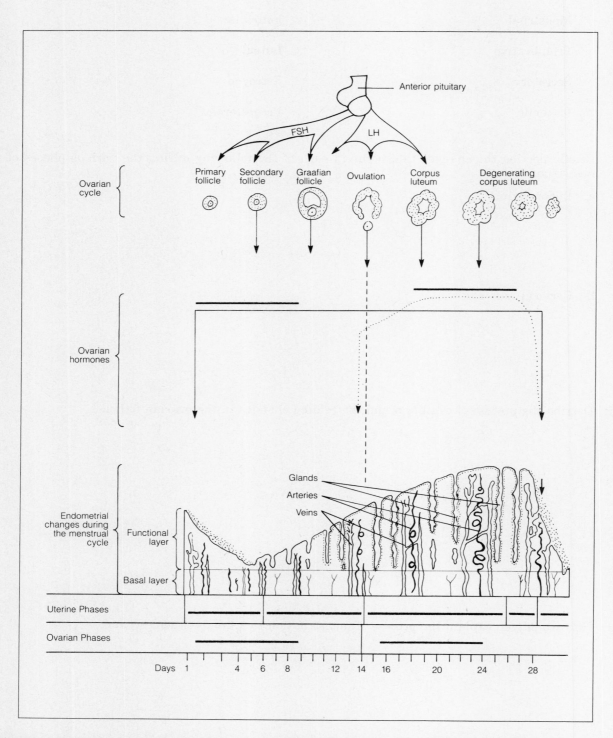

Figure 2–8 Female reproductive cycle: Interrelationships of hormones and the four phases of the uterine cycle and two phases of the ovarian cycle.

Infertility

37. Define the following terms:

    a. Infertility

    b. Primary infertility

    c. Secondary infertility

    d. Sterility

38. During a routine annual examination, your client tells you that she and her husband have been trying to conceive a child for about 8 months but have been unsuccessful. She asks you if there are any actions they can take to increase their chances of getting pregnant. What information would you give her?

39. Many factors in a woman's history may increase her risk of infertility. Identify at least five factors and briefly explain why they increase a woman's risk of infertility.

Factor	Influence on Fertility

40. Your client asks you about the use of basal body temperature (BBT) readings to identify ovulation.

    a. Describe the correct procedure for taking the BBT.

    b. Describe briefly the changes in temperature that will occur throughout a woman's cycle if she is ovulating.

41. Briefly discuss the emotional issues that a couple experiencing infertility may have.

42. For the following infertility tests, identify the purpose of the test and the procedure for completing the test.

Test	Purpose	Procedure
LH assay		
Progesterone assay		
Ultrasound		
Spinnbarkheit		
Ferning capacity		
Postcoital examination		
Hysterosalpingography		
Laparoscopy		

43. Discuss semen analysis as a diagnostic tool in an infertility workup. How is the semen collected? What findings indicate a normal semen analysis?

    A sperm count below _____ million/mL indicates probable infertility.

44. For each of the following medications used to treat infertility, summarize the purpose, method of administration, and possible side effects:

    a. Clomiphene citrate (Clomid)

    b. Human menopausal gonadotropin (hMG)

    c. Bromocriptine

    d. Gonadotropin-releasing hormone (GnRH)

45. Briefly describe the following reproductive technologies:

   a. Artificial insemination

   b. In vitro fertilization (IVF)

   c. Gamete intrafallopian transfer (GIFT)

   d. Zygote intrafallopian transfer (ZIFT)

*46. As a nurse working in an office that focuses on infertility evaluation and treatment, it is your responsibility to coordinate care for couples, provide ongoing information and teaching, and evaluate the couple's psychosocial status. Dorothy Lewis, age 37, has had extensive testing and treatment in an effort to correct her infertility, but all approaches have failed. During a conversation with you, Dorothy expresses the feeling that she is a failure as a woman and a wife. She states, "We both think that children are an important part of marriage, but because of me, because my body can't do what it should, we are the losers. I am such a failure as a woman." Based on this information, formulate a possible nursing diagnosis that might apply.

*47. Identify some of the defining characteristics that led you to the diagnosis.

---

*These questions are addressed at the end of Part I.

Genetic Disorders

48. How many chromosomes are found in a normal human somatic (body) cell? _____ .

    How many chromosomes are found in a sperm or an egg? _____ .

    The pictorial analysis of an individual's chromosomes is called a _____ .

49. Match the terms below with their correct definition:

    _____ Autosomal dominant inheritance

    a. Inherited disorder that manifests itself only as a homozygous trait

    _____ Autosomal recessive inheritance

    b. Inherited disorder that results from a combination of genetic and environmental factors

    _____ X-linked recessive inheritance

    c. Inherited disorder in which the disease trait is evident in heterozygous form

    _____ Multifactorial inheritance

    d. Inherited disorder in which the abnormal gene is carried on the X chromosome

*50. Your client's husband, who was adopted as an infant, has just been diagnosed as having Huntington's chorea. Your client asks you what the possibility is that their two children will develop the disease. What is the correct answer?

51. Diagram the pattern of inheritance demonstrating your rationale for your response.

*52. If one parent has cystic fibrosis and the other has normal genes, what is the probability that their children will have cystic fibrosis? Diagram your rationale for your response.

53. Draw a family tree (pedigree) for your family as far back as your grandparents if possible. Are there any conditions your family considers hereditary? Don't forget to include findings such as high blood pressure, obesity, and diabetes. If you are not familiar with drawing family trees (pedigrees) you may find it helpful to consult a physical assessment text.

Selected Answers

This section addresses the asterisked questions found in this chapter.

46. A possible nursing diagnosis that would apply is "Disturbance in self-esteem related to infertility." Depending on how successful the couple is in adjusting to the loss of the ability to conceive a child. Other nursing diagnoses that might apply are "Ineffective individual (or family) coping related to inability to accept infertility," or "Grieving related to loss of fertility" if the couple has made the decision to accept their childless status.

47. Defining characteristics that are present include
Negative body image (". . . my body can't do what it should.").
Low self-esteem (expressed feelings of failure).
Failure in role performance ("I am such a failure as a woman.").

50. Each child has a 50% chance of developing Huntington's chorea.

52. Because cystic fibrosis is an autosomal recessive disorder, an affected parent must have two genes for the disorder (that is, be homozygous). Thus, with one affected parent and one normal parent, none of the children would have the disorder, but all would be carriers of an abnormal gene for the disorder.

Part II Self-Assessment Guide

Do you know these abbreviations?

BBT	FRC	FSH
GnRH	GIFT	hCG
hMG	IVF	LH

Add your own abbreviations or new words you have learned:

Can you answer these questions?

The following multiple-choice questions will help you assess your knowledge of the content of this chapter. Select the best answer for each of the questions and then refer to the end of Part II to check your answers.

1. The ligaments that suspend the uterus from the lateral aspects of the true pelvis and provide the primary support for the uterus are the
    a. broad ligaments.
    b. cardinal ligaments.
    c. round ligaments.
    d. uterosacral ligaments.

2. What portion of the breast contains the cuboidal epithelial cells that secrete the components of milk?
    a. Alveoli
    b. Ducts
    c. Lactiferous sinuses
    d. Lobules

3. The figure-eight pattern of the middle layer of uterine muscle fibers
    a. constricts large uterine vessels when the fibers contract.
    b. differentiates the uterus into upper and lower segments.
    c. maintains the effects of uterine contractions during labor.
    d. maintains uterine shape during pregnancy.

A group of adolescents is waiting for pregnancy tests in a clinic. The nurse sees them talking and joins them to find out how much they know about the anatomy and physiology of their own bodies.

4. One of the girls asks about infections. The nurse explains that certain body functions protect the female from infection of the reproductive organs. Which of the following protects the female from infection of the reproductive organs?

   a. Alkaline pH and smegma secreted from the clitoris

   b. Acidic pH and bacteriostatic cervical mucosa

   c. Neutral pH of 7.5 and bactericidal secretions of labia minora

   d. pH of 4 to 5 and secretions of the Skene's ducts

5. One girl asks which hormone causes ovulation to occur. The nurse explains that about 18 hours after the peak production of _____ , ovulation occurs.

   a. Estrogen

   b. FSH (follicle-stimulating hormone)

   c. LH (luteinizing hormone)

   d. Progesterone

6. The nurse asks the girl to identify the hormone responsible for enhancing development of the graafian follicle and rebuilding the endometrium. The right answer would be

   a. estrogen.

   b. FSHRH (follicle-stimulating hormone–releasing hormone).

   c. GnRH (gonadotropin-releasing hormone).

   d. LHRH (luteinizing hormone–releasing hormone).

As the nurse leaves the clinic, the girl and her boyfriend approach and want to ask some questions. The nurse takes a deep breath and leans against the car in anticipation of their interest.

7. The girl then says she has one more question about the female cycle. She asks about the four phases of a single uterine cycle. Which of the four phases is eliminated if implantation occurs?

   a. Ischemic phase

   b. Menstrual phase

   c. Proliferative phase

   d. Secretory phase

8. Unlike the female ovaries, which are protected by lying deep inside the body, the male scrotum is outside the body. The teenagers ask why this is so. The most important purpose for the location of the scrotum is to

   a. maintain temperature lower than that of the body.

   b. produce sperm near the point of ejaculation.

   c. protect the testes and sperm from the effects of the prostate.

   d. provide room for the convoluted seminiferous tubules.

Jenny, age 14, approaches a nurse with questions about the physical changes occurring in some of her friends and people she knows. She says she's studying the reproductive system at school.

9. The onset of puberty occurs

    a. at approximately age 12 to 14, and it involves minor physical, psychologic, and emotional changes.

    b. over a period lasting from 1 1/2 to 5 years, and it results from the interaction of the central nervous system and the endocrine organs.

    c. slowly and earlier in boys than in girls.

    d. suddenly and earlier in girls than in boys.

10. The structure that provides a pathway for sperm to leave the epididymides is the

    a. dartos muscle.

    b. seminal vesicles.

    c. urethra.

    d. vas deferens.

11. Your client had a miscarriage two years ago. She and her partner have been trying to conceive a child for the past 18 months. Which of the following terms best describes her condition?

    a. Normal variation

    b. Primary infertility

    c. Secondary infertility

    d. Sterility

12. When monitoring basal body temperatures, which of the following patterns would indicate that ovulation had probably occurred?

    a. Temperature drops from 98.2°F to 97.8°F.

    b. Temperature increases from 97.4°F to 98.2°F and remains elevated.

    c. Temperature increases from 97.2°F to 97.6°F and then drops to 96.8°F.

    d. Temperature remains stable at 97.6°F.

13. The term *spinnbarkheit* refers to

    a. the changes in cervical mucus that occur throughout the ovulatory cycle.

    b. the distinct fern pattern of the cervical mucus at the time of ovulation.

    c. the increased elasticity of the cervical mucus at the time of ovulation.

    d. the midcycle or ovulatory pain some women experience.

14. A man with a sperm count of 53 million/mL

    a. has a borderline sperm count.

    b. has a normal sperm count.

    c. is considered infertile.

    d. is considered sterile.

15. Your client is a carrier of the X-linked disorder hemophilia. What is the statistical probability that any boys she gave birth to would have hemophilia?

    a. 25%

    b. 50%

    c. 75%

    d. 100%

16. Sickle cell anemia is an example of a/an

    a. autosomal, dominant, inherited disorder.

    b. autosomal, recessive, inherited disorder.

    c. multifactorial, inherited disorder.

    d. X-linked, recessive, inherited disorder.

Answers

1. b	2. a	3. a	4. b	5. c	6. a
7. a	8. a	9. b	10. d	11. c	12. b
13. c	14. b	15. b	16. b		

Women's Health Throughout the Life Span

3

Introduction

The woman of today has opportunities for personal and professional growth that did not exist 20 years ago. She also faces challenging social and health issues that influence her well-being and that of her family. A woman's health care needs change throughout her lifetime and may be influenced by a variety of factors, such as her age, her family history, her plans for childbearing, her sexual activity, and any abnormal findings that develop. This chapter focuses on selected social and health care issues, common breast disorders, and gynecologic problems. It concludes with a discussion of rape. It corresponds to Chapters 6, 7, 8, 9, and 10 in *Maternal-Newborn Nursing: A Family-Centered Approach,* 4th ed.

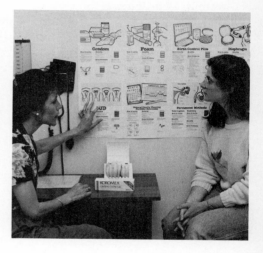

Part I Concepts, Critical Thinking, and Clinical Applications

Social Issues

1. Summarize the issues you think are most important for women today.

2. The phrase *feminization of poverty* has been used to describe the reality that many women live on incomes below poverty level. Discuss some of the factors that contribute to this phenomenon.

3. Maternity and/or paternity leave is under debate in the United States. List the advantages and disadvantages of having a leave policy.

4. Identify at least six workplace environmental hazards and state the risk they pose to the fetus if the woman is pregnant.

   a.

   b.

   c.

   d.

   e.

   f.

Human Sexuality

5. Identify the four phases of human sexual response described by Masters and Johnson.

   a.

   b.

   c.

   d.

6. Briefly describe the female and male sexual responses.

   a. Female

   b. Male

*7.   You have established a good relationship with a 14-year-old girl who is seen at the family practice clinic where you work. One day she says, "My sister told me that when I get turned on by a guy, I'll find myself getting wet between my legs. Is that true? Why does that happen?" How would you respond?

*8.   A 26-year-old woman tells you that occasionally when she and her husband make love in the morning it is painful for her. She says, "Since I work nights and he works days, it is pretty rushed. I'm exhausted and ready to sleep while he's hurrying because he has to get to work. Sometimes I'm hardly lubricated and I don't feel aroused at all. Then it feels as though he's crashing into something inside me each time he thrusts. That really hurts. What's happening?"

The Role of the Nurse in Menstrual Counseling

*9.   You are teaching girls 11 to 12 years of age about self-care during menstruation. What topics would you discuss with these girls?

10.   Discuss premenstrual syndrome (PMS) with regard to etiology, signs and symptoms, and treatment. Include information on self-care measures women with PMS might employ.

11.   Match the definitions listed on the right with the correct terms below.

Term	Definition
_____ Amenorrhea	a. Abnormally short menstrual cycle
_____ Hypomenorrhea	b. Absence of menses
_____ Menorrhagia	c. Excessive menstrual flow
_____ Dysmenorrhea	d. Bleeding between periods
_____ Hypermenorrhea	e. Painful menses
_____ Metrorrhagia	f. Abnormally long menstrual cycle

*These questions are addressed at the end of Part I.

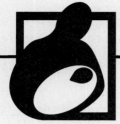

It's Your Turn

Some women view menstruation as a normal, even welcome, part of life; some women view it as a minor annoyance; some women are embarrassed by it; others consider it a "curse" and hate it. These attitudes are influenced by a variety of factors. Take a few moments to explore your views on menstruation. Try to identify some of the factors that have influenced your beliefs about it.

_____

_____

_____

_____

_____

_____

_____

_____

_____

_____

_____

_____

_____

_____

_____

_____

Contraceptive Methods

12. You are discussing contraception with a group of women. Complete the following chart:

Contraceptive Method	Mechanism of Action	Side Effects/ Untoward Effects	Patient Teaching
Oral contraceptives Reliability _____			
Intrauterine device Reliability _____			
Norplant® Reliability _____			
Diaphragm Reliability _____			
Cervical cap Reliability _____			
Foams, jellies, film, vaginal suppositories, and condoms Reliability _____			
Fertility awareness methods Reliability _____			
Coitus interruptus Reliability _____			
Postcoital douche Reliability _____			

Menopause

*13. Mrs Joan Sanchez, age 50, has been coming to this office for her gynecologic exams for the past seven years. Last year, she mentioned some irregularity in her periods. During her annual physical exam and Pap smear, she tells you that her periods have been more irregular and her last period was about three months ago. In addition, she has been experiencing difficulty sleeping; a sense of heat rising over her chest, neck, and face; increased perspiration; and palpitations. You identify that Mrs. Sanchez is entering menopause. In your counseling session, what information about self-care measures can you provide?

*14. The following situation has been included to challenge your critical thinking. Read the situation and then answer the question "yes" or "no." Yvonne Swenson, age 52, is being seen for her annual examination. Her history reveals that she is a slender woman of Swedish ancestry who completed menopause at age 46. She does not drink alcohol but does smoke three-fourths of a pack of cigarettes per day. She has two children.

Is Ms Swenson at increased risk of developing osteoporosis? _____

⇓ ⇓

Yes (Why? _____) No (Why not? _____)

*15. In women who have a uterus and who are on hormone replacement therapy (HRT), the estrogen is

opposed by giving _____ for all or part of the cycle to prevent the increased

risk of developing _____ .

---

*These questions are addressed at the end of Part I.

The Female Breast

16. Identify common signs of fibrocystic breast disease.

*17. Your client asks if there are any self-care measures she can use to attempt to decrease the discomfort she experiences cyclically because of fibrocystic breast disease. What advice would you give her?

18. Pretend you are responsible for teaching the correct procedure for monthly breast self-examination to healthy women.

   *a. Explain the purpose for visually inspecting the breasts with the arms in a variety of positions.

   b. What findings would be considered abnormal on inspection?

   c. How would you explain the procedure for palpating the breasts and axillae?

19. For each of the following surgical procedures used in the treatment of cancer of the breast, describe the extent of the procedure and identify the rationale for its use.

    a. Radical mastectomy

    b. Modified radical mastectomy

    c. Total (simple) mastectomy

    d. Subcutaneous mastectomy

    e. Partial (segmental) mastectomy

    f. Wide local excision (lumpectomy)

20. Briefly discuss the value of reconstructive surgery and identify women who are good candidates for the procedure.

*21. Valerie Petropoulis was recently diagnosed as having early breast cancer and is evaluating her treatment options. Identify at least three nursing diagnoses that may apply at this time.

a.

b.

c.

22. Describe briefly the nurse's role in caring for a woman with breast cancer during the

a. Diagnostic period

b. Preoperative period

c. Postoperative period

23. The three most common symptoms of endometriosis are

    a.

    b.

    c.

*24. In the office where you work as a nurse, one of the women being treated for endometriosis is going to begin taking danazol. You assess her knowledge level and find that she has only a vague understanding of the medication. You formulate the nursing diagnosis: Knowledge deficit related to the medication danazol. Based on this nursing diagnosis, what information would you give her about the drug?

25. Your client asks you about health practices she can follow to help her avoid developing toxic shock syndrome. What recommendations would you make?

26. For each of the infections listed in the first column (on the next page), identify the causative organism, common signs and symptoms, method of diagnosis, medical therapy, and appropriate health teaching to help prevent the spread or relieve discomfort.

---

*These questions are addressed at the end of Part I.

Infection	Causative Organism	Signs	Diagnosis	Therapy	Teaching
Moniliasis					
Bacterial vaginosis					
Trichomoniasis					
Chlamydia					
Herpes genitalis					
Syphilis					
Gonorrhea					
Condyloma accuminata					
Pediculosis pubis					
Scabies					

The following action sequence is designed to help you think through clinical problems. We've answered portions of it at the end of Part I.

*27. **Action Sequence**
   Pretend you work as a registered nurse in a women's health clinic. It is your responsibility to interview women initially and obtain data on the purpose of their visit. You also do health teaching. You do not do pelvic examinations. Nita Trujillo, a client at the clinic, tells you that she is there today because she has had marked itching of her vulva and vagina. She states, "It itches so bad that I've scratched it raw and made it worse." She tells you she has never had a vaginal infection before and has not been sexually active for 3 months. She says that she has had no symptoms of a urinary tract infection although it does burn when the urine touches the excoriated skin.

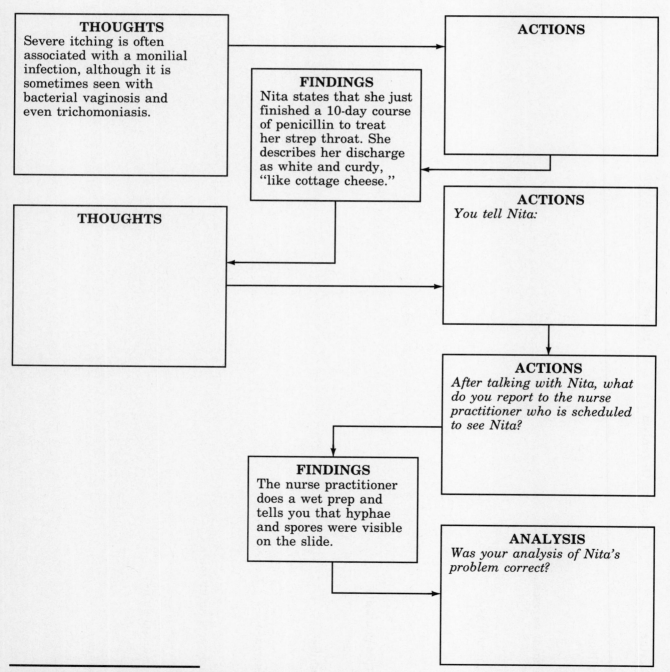

THOUGHTS
Severe itching is often associated with a monilial infection, although it is sometimes seen with bacterial vaginosis and even trichomoniasis.

FINDINGS
Nita states that she just finished a 10-day course of penicillin to treat her strep throat. She describes her discharge as white and curdy, "like cottage cheese."

ACTIONS

THOUGHTS

ACTIONS
You tell Nita:

ACTIONS
After talking with Nita, what do you report to the nurse practitioner who is scheduled to see Nita?

FINDINGS
The nurse practitioner does a wet prep and tells you that hyphae and spores were visible on the slide.

ANALYSIS
Was your analysis of Nita's problem correct?

28. Compare cystitis and pyelonephritis:

	Cystitis	Pyelonephritis
Signs and symptoms		
Therapy		
Implications		
Client education		

Gynecologic Surgery

29. Your client asks you why some women have an abdominal hysterectomy while others have a vaginal hysterectomy. How would you respond?

30. You are a nurse working on a gynecologic surgery unit where you often care for women following hysterectomies. Outline the information that should be included for women as part of discharge teaching.

31. List at least five indications for performing a dilation and curettage (D & C).

    a.

    b.

    c.

    d.

    e.

32. Briefly summarize the physiologic implications for a premenopausal woman when both ovaries are surgically removed (oophorectomy).

33. For each of the following procedures, identify the purpose and briefly describe the process by which the procedure is done:

Procedure	Purpose	Process
Colposcopy		
Biopsy		
Conization		
Cryosurgery		
Laser therapy		

34. Briefly summarize the treatment alternatives available to a woman with cancer of the cervix.

The Crisis of Rape

35. Define *rape*.

36. Identify the four stages of a victim's crisis response to rape:

    a.

    b.

    c.

    d.

37. The nursing diagnosis "Rape trauma syndrome" is a broad and yet specific diagnosis that can be used without the phrase *related to*. For this diagnosis, identify the defining characteristics that may be present during the acute phase.

38. Identify actions the nurse might take to assist a woman who has been raped to cope with the acute phase of the rape trauma syndrome.

Selected Answers

This section addresses the asterisked questions found in this chapter.

7. Adolescents have many questions about their own sexuality and often are surprisingly uninformed. We hope you will explain that her body will prepare itself to enjoy lovemaking. This preparation begins with aroused feelings, perhaps due to kissing, touching, or exchanging loving words with her partner. You can explain that the "wetness" is due to the seeping of fluids (transudation) along her vagina. The fluid serves as a lubricant so that if lovemaking occurs, it is smooth and pleasurable. You can also explain other physical and emotional changes that occur during the sexual reponse cycle. It may be helpful to give her a chance to ask more questions, since she seems to trust you.

8. This woman's discomfort is probably related to inadequate arousal, for when a woman is aroused, the transudation of fluids lubricates her vagina. In addition, her uterus draws up and back so that the vagina lengthens to accommodate the erect penis. Without this arousal, the lengthening doesn't occur. Her discomfort results from the force of her husband's thrust against her cervix and from friction because of inadequate lubrication. We hope that after you explain this to her, you will explore with her ways to improve her situation. She needs to share this information with her husband so they can plan to allow more time for foreplay. It may be necessary to find a different time for lovemaking—perhaps in early evening when they are both rested.

9. Menstrual self-care measures you could discuss with the girls include sanitary protection measures (tampons, sanitary pads); vaginal deodorant sprays; general cleanliness measures; and the impact of measures such as exercise, diet, and heat on menstrual discomfort (cramping). This information may help young girls gain a positive attitude toward the menstrual experience.

13. Information Mrs Sanchez would benefit from includes the following self-care measures: the use of a fan and/or increased intake of cold liquids for the hot flashes, continued calcium supplementation, and use of water-soluble jelly during intercourse to counteract vaginal atrophy (increased frequency of intercourse also will maintain some elasticity in the vagina if this is an area of concern for her). It may also be of value to Mrs Sanchez to discuss other physical and emotional responses that may occur in menopause.

14. If you answered "yes," you are right. Congratulations. Ms Swenson has several factors that place her at increased risk for osteoporosis, including early onset of menopause, fair complexion, slender build, and history of smoking.

15. In HRT the estrogen is opposed by progesterone, usually Provera, to prevent endometrial hyperplasia, which increases the risk of endometrial cancer.

17. You would probably mention simple practices such as limiting sodium intake and wearing a supportive bra. If the discomfort is especially severe, the woman may ask her care giver for a prescription for a mild diuretic and might also use a nonprescription analgesic. Even though the data regarding the value of limiting methylxanthines (found in caffeine products) is controversial, it can't hurt, and many women feel it is helpful. If you give the woman this information, she can then choose whether she wishes to try it. You can also mention that some people feel thiamine and vitamin E are helpful, although this has not been supported by clinical research. When you share this information honestly, you enable the woman to make her own health care choices based on available information. Use this time to stress the importance of monthly breast self-examination and regular mammograms as recommended by her health care provider.

18. a. It is helpful to point out that all women have breasts that vary slightly in size and contour, but inspection helps a woman to know her own breasts so that she can recognize changes. Changes in the way her breasts move or point as she moves her arms through a variety of positions can be significant. Moving the arms through a variety of positions also varies the pull on the skin and muscles of the chest so that masses or changes that are not visible in one position may become evident in another position.

21. Many nursing diagnoses may apply to Valerie Petropoulis as she evaluates her treatment options. The following are a few possibilities:

    a. Decisional conflict about treatment options related to lack of detailed information.

    b. Fear related to diagnosis of breast cancer.

    c. Body image disturbance related to expressed fear of disfigurement secondary to surgery.

    d. Knowledge deficit related to confusion about treatment alternatives.

    Other diagnoses that may apply include ineffective family coping, ineffective individual coping, anticipatory grieving, situational low self-esteem, and so forth.

24. We hope you would discuss her medication in detail with her. It is important to review the purpose of the medication and possible side effects. You should also be certain that she clearly understands the dosage and administration schedule. In many instances women take danazol for a specified period of time (from three months to eight months or longer), depending on the severity of the disease and the presence of palpable lesions. If she is scheduled to return for reevaluation at specified times, it is important that she understand the purpose and significance of these evaluations. Answer any questions she might have and give her an opportunity to voice any concerns about the therapy. If this medication is prescribed frequently in your office, you may want to develop a handout on it for clients to refer to when they are at home.

27. *Actions:* In making your assessment it would be helpful to ask Nita whether she has noticed any change in her vaginal discharge. If she has, ask her to describe it. Because of the relationship between antibiotic therapy and monilial infection, you would ask whether she had been on antibiotics for any reason. It is always useful to ask clients whether they attribute the symptoms to anything. You may gain useful information about the condition or information about the client's perceptions.

    Thoughts: Based on the information obtained, you suspect that Nita has monilial vaginitis.

    Actions: You tell Nita that, based on her symptoms, you suspect that she may have a yeast infection called monilial vaginitis. You point out that sometimes when women take antibiotics to destroy a bacterial infection, the antibiotics also destroy the normal, good bacteria found in a woman's vagina. When this happens, other organisms, especially yeast, may grow unchecked. You tell Nita that you will report your findings to the nurse-practitioner (NP). You point out that the NP will probably do a vaginal examination and a test to confirm the infection type.

Actions: You would briefly describe Nita's symptoms and the appearance of her vaginal discharge and report the recent antibiotic therapy. You would say that you suspect that Nita might have a monilial infection and ask the NP if she planned to do a vaginal examination and wet prep.

Analysis: Congratulations! Your analysis of the data was accurate. Hyphae and spores indicate monilial infection. Give yourself a pat on the back, too, for working in a collegial fashion with the NP.

Part II Self-Assessment Guide

Do you know these abbreviations?

BBT	BSE
CDC	D & C
FBD	PID
STD	UTI

Add your own abbreviations or new words you have learned:

Can you answer these questions?

The following multiple-choice questions will help you assess your knowledge of the content of this chapter. Select the best answer for each of the questions and then refer to the end of Part II to check your answers.

1. Which of the following events occurs during the plateau stage of the female sexual response?
    a. Nipples become erect.
    b. Orgasmic platform develops.
    c. Uterus contracts rhythmically.
    d. Vaginal lubrication appears.

2. In reviewing a chart you learn that your client has a history of dysmenorrhea. This means that she has
    a. bleeding between menstrual cycles.
    b. excessively heavy menstrual flow.
    c. irregular menstrual cycles.
    d. painful menstrual periods.

3. What is the mechanism of action of Norplant®?
    a. It creates thin, watery cervical mucus.
    b. It destroys sperm.
    c. It prevents implantation.
    d. It prevents ovulation.

4. Which of the following is a risk factor for osteoporosis?
   a. Black race
   b. Late onset of menopause
   c. Multiparity
   d. Thin and small-boned

5. Which of the following findings during breast self-examination should a woman report to her health care provider?
   a. Difference in size between the breasts
   b. Silver colored striae
   c. Symmetrical venous pattern
   d. Thickened skin with enlarged pores

6. A primary side effect of danazol (Danocrine) is
   a. dry, flaky skin.
   b. hirsutism.
   c. increased libido.
   d. weight loss.

7. Which of the following women has the greatest risk of breast cancer?
   a. 26-year-old female with high-protein, high-fat diet
   b. 52-year-old female whose mother and sister died of breast cancer
   c. 43-year-old unmarried female whose menarche occurred at age 14
   d. 35-year-old upper-middle-class female with slightly cystic breasts

8. The presence of clue cells on a wet mount preparation is indicative of
   a. bacterial vaginosis.
   b. *Candida albicans.*
   c. chlamydia.
   d. trichomoniasis.

9. Which of the following medications may be used in the treatment of condyloma accuminata?
   a. Acyclovir
   b. Metronidazole
   c. Miconazole
   d. Podophyllin

10. Which of the following is indicative of a lower urinary tract infection (cystitis)?
    a. Dysuria
    b. Flank pain
    c. Glycosuria
    d. High fever

Answers

1. b   2. d   3. d   4. d   5. d   6. b   7. b   8. a   9. d   10. a

Conception and Fetal Development

4

Introduction

The conception and development of a new human being is a never-ending source of awe and fascination. As our knowledge of this process evolves, we develop greater insight into the potential ramifications of the physiologic, psychologic, and environmental factors that may impinge on it.

This chapter begins with a review of the process of conception. It then considers implantation, placental functioning, and fetal development. Factors that may influence fetal development are explored, with special emphasis on the impact of maternal medications.

This chapter's strong emphasis on anatomy and physiology provides a basis for subsequent chapters on the application of the nursing process for a childbearing family and corresponds to Chapter 11 in *Maternal-Newborn Nursing: A Family-Centered Approach,* 4th ed.

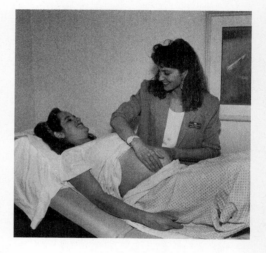

Part I Concepts, Critical Thinking, and Clinical Applications

1. As a review, match the following terms with the appropriate description:

   a. Genes _____ Structures made up of DNA strands and proteins

   b. Chromosomes _____ Germ cells containing the haploid number (23) of chromosomes

   c. Sex chromosomes _____ Areas on DNA strands that determine each individual's characteristics

   d. Gametes _____ The 23rd pair of chromosomes, either XX or XY

2. Briefly compare mitosis and meiosis.

3. Each sperm and ovum has _____ chromosomes.

4. The normal newborn has _____ chromosomes.

5. The _____ chromosome determines the sex of the child and the _____ carries this chromosome.

6. The optimal place for fertilization to occur is in the _____ , and it needs to occur _____ hours after ovulation of the ovum and _____ hours after ejaculation.

7. Briefly describe the process of fertilization.

8. What two processes must the sperm undergo in order to fertilize the ovum?

   a.

   b.

9. What mechanism(s) is(are) involved in transporting the zygote (fertilized ovum) from the fallopian tube to the uterus?

10. The zygote continually develops as it travels through the fallopian tube to its site of implantation in the uterus. Match each of the following terms with the appropriate description.

    a. Cleavage   _____ Period of rapid cellular division

    b. Blastomeres   _____ Outer layer of cells that replaces the zona pellucida

    c. Morula   _____ Small developing mass of cells held together by zona pellucida

    d. Blastocyst   _____ Solid ball of cells

    e. Trophoblasts   _____ Inner solid mass of cells after cavity has formed

11. Implantation occurs about _____ to _____ days after fertilization.

12. Briefly describe how implantation occurs.

13. Define the following terms related to the endometrium after implantation:
   a. Decidua

   b. Decidua capsularis

   c. Decidua basalis

   d. Decidua vera (parietalis)

Embryonic Membranes/Amniotic Fluid

14. The embryonic membranes begin to form at the time of implantation. Two distinct membranes develop, the _____ and the _____ .

15. Describe the normal amount and composition of amniotic fluid.

16. List three functions of amniotic fluid.

    a.

    b.

    c.

17. Describe the following stages of human development in utero.

    a. Embryo

    b. Fetus

18. Using your answers to questions 13, 14, and 17, fill in the blanks on Figure 4–1, the early development of the baby.

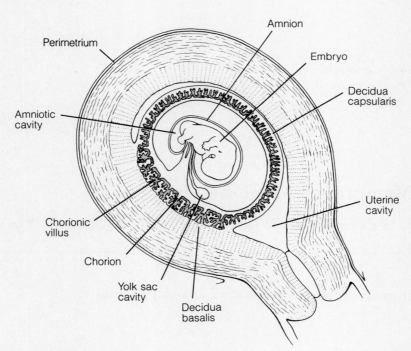

Figure 4–1 Early development of the baby. This figure depicts early development of selected structures at approximately eight weeks. (From Spence AP, Mason EB: *Human Anatomy and Physiology,* 3rd ed. Menlo Park, CA: Benjamin/Cummings Pub. Co., 1987, p 851)

19. Identify the three primary germ layers of the developing fetus and at least two structures derived from each layer.

Germ Layer	Developing Structures
a.	
b.	
c.	

20. Briefly describe the process by which the placenta develops and its component structures.

21. Describe how the appearance of the maternal side of the placenta differs from the appearance of the fetal side.

22. Identify three major functions of the placenta.

    a.

    b.

    c.

23. List the four major placental hormones and their function during pregnancy.

Hormone	Function
a.	
b.	
c.	
d.	

*24. Describe the visual assessments you would want to make of the placenta after birth.

Fetal Circulation

25. The body stalk, which attaches the embryo to the yolk sac, will develop into the umbilical cord. The umbilical cord is made up of _____ vein(s), _____ artery(ies), and specialized connective tissue called _____ whose function is to _____ .

26. Circle the answer that correctly completes these sentences.

    The umbilical vein carries (**oxygenated**) or (**deoxygenated**) blood (**to**) or (**away from**) the fetus. The umbilical arteries carry (**oxygenated**) or (**deoxygenated**) blood (**from**) or (**to**) the fetus to the placenta.

---

*These questions are addressed at the end of Part I.

27. Label the following structures on Figure 4–2 and, using arrows, trace the normal pathway of fetal circulation:

Umbilical vein

Foramen ovale

Ductus venosus

Ductus arteriosus

Inferior vena cava

Umbilical arteries

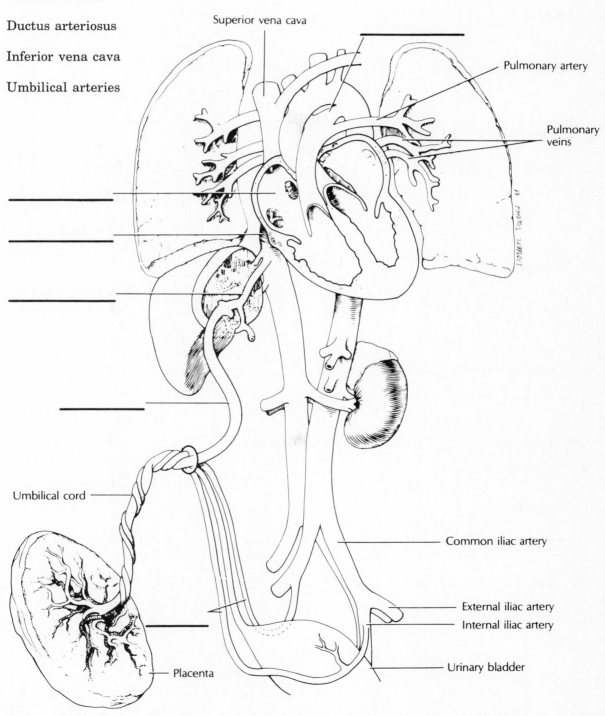

Figure 4–2   Fetal circulation (From Spence, AP, Mason, EB: *Human Anatomy and Physiology.* 3rd. ed. Menlo Park, CA: Benjamin/Cummings Pub. Co., 1987, p 862.)

28. Describe the function of each of the following fetal structures during fetal life and the changes that occur after birth.

	Fetal*	Newborn
a. Umbilical vein		
b. Ductus venosus		
c. Inferior vena cava		
d. Foramen ovale		
e. Ductus arteriosus		
f. Umbilical arteries		

*These questions are addressed at the end of Part I.

29. Complete the following chart of embryonic and fetal development.

Gestational Age	Length	Weight	Anatomic/Physiologic Developmental Characteristics
4 weeks			
8 weeks			
12 weeks			
16 weeks			
20 weeks			
24 weeks			
28 weeks			
36 weeks			

*30. Identify four factors that influence embryonic and fetal development.

   a.

   b.

   c.

   d.

31. The fetus is most vulnerable to congenital malformation development during the first _____ weeks of life.

32. You are assisting in a prenatal class on fetal development. Mrs Elizabeth Oliver, a 22-year-old primigravida, is 14 weeks pregnant and has the following questions. Based on your knowledge of fetal development, how would you respond?

   a. "When will my baby look like a baby?"

   b. "How long is my baby now and how much does it weigh?"

   c. "When will I feel my baby move?"

   d. "When will my baby's heart start beating?"

   e. "When can my baby's sex be identified?"

   f. "Can my baby open its eyes?"

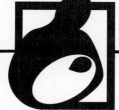

It's Your Turn

Feeling movement brings images of the future baby to moms and dads. What have parents told you about this, or what have you personally felt?

_____

_____

_____

_____

_____

_____

_____

_____

_____

_____

_____

Selected Answers

This section addresses the asterisked questions found in this chapter.

24. The significant observations that you would want to make about the placenta would include determining the presence of all cotyledons, the presence of large infarcts or clots in the placenta, and the site of the umbilical insertion on the placenta. These observations will give you clues to potential problems for the newborn. The absence of cotyledons would indicate a need to have the clinician check the mother for retained placental fragments that could cause postpartum hemorrhage later.

28. Fetal circulation differs significantly from infant and adult circulation in that the fetus's oxygenated blood originates from the placenta and flows into the right atrium. It then moves through the foramen ovale (because of the low resistance on the left side of the fetal heart) and out the aorta to provide the head and upper body with highly oxygenated blood. Very little oxygenated blood flows into the lungs because they are collapsed and offer a high resistance to blood flow. The blood that goes through the pulmonary artery is shunted into the aorta through the ductus arteriosus, bypassing the lungs to supply the rest of the body.

30. Many factors can influence the development of the embyro or fetus. Significant ones include the quality of the sperm or ova, teratogenic agents such as drugs and radiation, and maternal nutrition. Others you might have identified are any of the complications of pregnancy, such as maternal diabetes, hypertension, or TORCH infections.

Part II Self-Assessment Guide

Do you know these abbreviations?

AF   hCS   hPL

Add your own abbreviations or new words that you have learned:

Can you answer these questions?

The following multiple-choice questions will help you assess your knowledge of the content of this chapter. Select the best answer for each of the questions and then refer to the end of Part II to check your answers.

The nurse in a large prenatal clinic is conducting classes on pregnancy for 12 couples from the local university. This class explores conception and the development of the fetus.

1. The nurse tells the couples that fertilization occurs in the
    a. cervix.
    b. fallopian tube.
    c. ovary.
    d. uterus.

2. "I have a question about how long the egg and the sperm live," Joe asks. The nurse answers that, once released, the ovum remains fertile for _____ hours, while the ejaculated sperm lives for _____ day(s).
    a. 2 to 12; 1
    b. 6 to 24; 2 to 3
    c. 36 to 48; 4 to 10
    d. 72 to 96; 38 to 42

3. A client asks how long it takes the fertilized egg to attach to the uterus. The nurse replies that implantation occurs about _____ hours/days after fertilization:
    a. 1 to 2 hours
    b. 12 to 24 hours
    c. 3 to 5 days
    d. 7 to 9 days

4. "Can you tell us about the baby's heart?" Linda replies, "The heart of the embryo is a distinguishable organ by the _____ week of development."
    a. 8th
    b. 14th
    c. 17th
    d. 24th

5. The morula, or "mulberry mass," is

   a. a small ball of cells.

   b. layers of cells surrounding a fluid-filled sac.

   c. the differentiation of primary germ layers.

   d. the outer layer of cells replacing the zona pellucida.

6. The chorion is

   a. a thick membrane that develops from trophoblasts.

   b. a thin protective membrane containing amniotic fluid.

   c. the endometrium after implantation.

   d. the second cavity in the blastocyst.

7. A client asks, "What prevents intrauterine compression of the umbilical cord and its blood vessels?" The nurse explains that intrauterine compression of the umbilical cord is prevented by

   a. a cushion of amniotic fluid.

   b. a thick muscle layer.

   c. connective tissue known as Wharton's jelly, plus high blood volume pulsating through the vessels.

   d. highly absorbent vessel walls.

8. The mesoderm germ layer gives rise to the following structures:

   a. Alimentary canal, lungs, liver, and bladder

   b. Circulatory system, skin epithelium, and reproductive organs

   c. Muscles, lungs, and circulatory system

   d. Nervous system, lungs, and genitourinary system

9. At term, the placenta is

   a. 2–4 inches in diameter and 1 inch thick at the center and weighs 1/5 of the weight of the newborn.

   b. 6–8 inches in diameter and 1 inch thick and composed of 5–10 cotyledons.

   c. composed of 10–15 cotyledons and 6–8 inches in diameter and 1/2 inch thick in the center.

   d. composed of 15–20 cotyledons and weighs approximately 1/6 of the weight of the newborn.

10. The placenta produces which hormone to maintain pregnancy?

   a. Estrogen

   b. Luteinizing hormone

   c. Progesterone

   d. Testosterone

11. The fetal sex organs have differentiated and are developed by the end of the

   a. first lunar month.

   b. second lunar month.

   c. third lunar month.

   d. fourth lunar month.

12. A fetus weighing about 300 gm and measuring 18 cm in length that can actively suck and swallow amniotic fluid is approximately how many weeks gestation?

    a. 14 weeks

    b. 18 weeks

    c. 20 weeks

    d. 24 weeks

Susan Tyler is in her 37th week of pregnancy. She has been seen on a regular basis and has been receptive to medical and nursing recommendations.

13. Susan confides that she tried some marijuana at a friend's house recently. She asks about the effect the drug will have on her baby. Which of the following statements is true?

    a. An injurious agent has the greatest effect on the cells that are growing the most rapidly.

    b. Susan's baby will most likely experience brain damage as a result of this teratogen.

    c. The most critical time in Susan's pregnancy for fetal damage from teratogenic drugs is 38 to 40 weeks.

    d. When taken in any amount or at any time in the pregnancy, marijuana will probably not result in any harmful effects.

14. At 37 weeks, Susan's baby is most likely

    a. depositing layers of subcutaneous fat.

    b. developing hair and fingernails.

    c. storing vitamins and minerals for future brain growth.

    d. thickening skin layers for thermal insulation.

Answers

1. b	2. b	3. d	4. a	5. a	6. a	7. c
8. c	9. d	10. c	11. b	12. c	13. a	14. a

Physical and Psychologic Changes of Pregnancy

5

Introduction

During pregnancy, a woman's body undergoes a variety of changes designed to facilitate the growth and optimal maintenance of her developing fetus. Although the changes in her reproductive tract are the most dramatic, virtually all systems of her body are affected. In addition to physical changes, major psychologic changes occur as the couple adjusts to the fact that they will soon be parents.

This chapter focuses on the physical and psychologic changes that occur in preparation for childbirth. Subsequent chapters explore the nursing assessments and interventions that should accompany these changes. This chapter corresponds to Chapter 12 in *Maternal-Newborn Nursing: A Family-Centered Approach*, 4th ed.

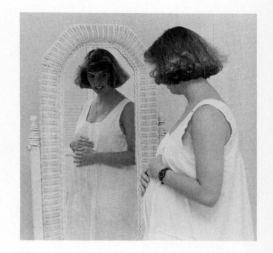

Part I Concepts, Critical Thinking, and Clinical Applications

Anatomy and Physiology of Pregnancy

1. Briefly describe changes in the size of the uterus that occur as a result of pregnancy.

2. Identify the major factors that contribute to the dramatic increase in uterine size.

3. How are the circulatory requirements of the uterus affected by pregnancy?

4. Many of the changes that occur in the pelvic organs during pregnancy are named. For each of the following changes, identify its correct name:

   a. The deep reddish-purple coloration of the mucosa of the cervix, vagina, and vulva is called

      _____ sign.

   b. The softening of the cervix that occurs is called _____ sign.

   c. The softening of the isthmus of the uterus is called _____ sign.

5. How is the mucous plug formed? What is its function?

6. The ovaries _____ ovum production during pregnancy.

7. What is the effect of pregnancy on the corpus luteum?

8. What is the significance of the increased acidity of the vaginal secretions during pregnancy?

9. Describe the breast changes that occur during pregnancy with regard to the following:

   a. Size

   b. Pigmentation

   c. Montgomery's tubercles

   d. Formation and appearance of striae gravidarum

   e. Sensation

10. a. What is colostrum?

    b. When does colostrum generally appear?

11. Why is there an increased tendency toward nasal stuffiness and epistaxis during pregnancy?

12. Briefly describe the changes that occur in the respiratory system during pregnancy.

13. How are the following components of the cardiovascular system affected by pregnancy?
    a. Blood volume

    b. Pulse rate

    c. Hemoglobin concentration

14. Explain the pseudoanemia frequently seen in pregnancy.

15. During pregnancy, the enlarging uterus may cause pressure on the vena cava when the woman lies supine, interfering with returning blood flow. As a result the woman may feel dizzy and clammy, and her blood pressure may decrease. This condition is called the _____ syndrome or _____ syndrome.

16. What is the cause of "heartburn" during pregnancy?

17. Why do bloating and constipation occur during pregnancy?

18. Explain why hemorrhoids often develop during pregnancy.

19. What effect does the growing uterus have on the bladder?

20. What is the significance of the increase in the glomerular filtration rate that occurs during pregnancy?

21. Many changes occur in the skin during pregnancy. Match the terms identifying these changes with their appropriate definition:

_____ Chloasma

_____ Striae gravidarum

_____ Spider nevi

_____ Linea nigra

a. Line of darker pigmentation extending from the pubis to the umbilicus in some women

b. Small, bright red, vascular elevations of the skin often found on the chest, arms, legs, and neck

c. The "mask of pregnancy," an irregular pigmentation commonly found on the cheeks, forehead, and nose

d. Wavy, irregular, reddish streaks commonly found on the abdomen, breasts, or thighs; often referred to as "stretch marks"

*22. A pregnant woman tells you that her friends tease her about her "stomach-first, waddling walk." She asks why she walks this way. How would you respond?

23. Briefly describe the functions of the following hormones in pregnancy:

a. Human chorionic gonadotropin (hCG)

b. Estrogen

c. Progesterone

d. Human placental lactogen (hPL)

e. Relaxin

24. Briefly discuss the influence of prostaglandins on pregnancy.

25. Describe the effects of pregnancy on the following components of the endocrine system:

    a. Thyroid

    b. Parathyroid

    c. Pituitary

    d. Adrenals

26. What is the average weight gain during each trimester of pregnancy?

    a. First trimester:

    b. Second trimester:

    c. Third trimester:

27. Why does water retention commonly occur during pregnancy?

28. How is the metabolism of the following substances affected by pregnancy?

    a. Protein

    b. Carbohydrates

    c. Fats

    d. Minerals

29. Indicate when the following signs of pregnancy occur and identify them as subjective (presumptive), objective (probable), or diagnostic (positive). For the signs that are subjective or objective, indicate other causative factors.

	Time of Appearance	Subjective (Presump-tive)	Objective (Probable)	Diagnostic (Positive)	Other Causative Factors
Enlarging abdomen					
Goodell's sign					
Braxton Hicks contractions					
Fetal heart sounds					
Excessive fatigue					
Positive pregnancy test					
Nausea and vomiting					
Urinary frequency					
Breast changes					
Fetal movements					
Chadwick's sign					

	Time of Appearance	Subjective (Presumptive)	Objective (Probable)	Diagnostic (Positive)	Other Causative Factors
Skin pigmentation changes					
Hegar's sign					
Amenorrhea					
Quickening					
Ladin's sign					

30. How would you explain the differences among subjective (presumptive), objective (probable), and diagnostic (positive) signs of pregnancy to an expectant mother?

Pregnancy Tests

31. Briefly describe each of the following pregnancy tests:

   Immunoassay

   a. Agglutination-inhibition test (Pregnosticon R)

   b. Latex agglutination tests (Gravindex and Pregnosticon slide test)

   c. Beta subunit radioimmunoassay (hCG and Preg/Stat β-hCG)

   d. Enzyme-linked immunosorbent assay (ELISA)

Radioreceptor Assay

a. Radioreceptor assay (Biocept G)

32. What factors may influence the reliability of a pregnancy test?

33. Why is a positive pregnancy test *not* a positive sign of pregnancy?

*34. What factors contribute to false readings in using over-the-counter pregnancy tests?

---

*These questions are addressed at the end of Part I.

Psychologic Response of the Expectant Family to Pregnancy

35. Briefly summarize behaviors that are commonly seen in each trimester as a woman adjusts to pregnancy.

Trimester	Behaviors
First trimester	
Second trimester	
Third trimester	

*36. Discuss the possible effects of pregnancy on a woman's body image.

---

*37. Rubin (1984) suggests that a pregnant woman faces four main psychologic tasks as she works to maintain her intactness and that of her family while also preparing a place for her new child. Identify and briefly summarize these tasks.

a.

b.

c.

d.

*38. Your close friend has just received confirmation that she is 10 weeks pregnant. She tells you that she feels some ambivalence about being pregnant and having a child, even though the pregnancy was planned. How might you respond?

---

*These questions are addressed at the end of Part I.

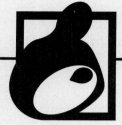

It's Your Turn

Think of some pregnant women you have known or cared for who were
at different stages of pregnancy. How did their responses to pregnancy
vary? What feelings did they describe? How did their partners react?
Their parents? Other children in the family?

_____

_____

_____

_____

_____

_____

_____

_____

_____

_____

_____

_____

_____

_____

_____

_____

_____

39. Discuss the reactions of expectant fathers to pregnancy with regard to the following:

    a. Role change

    b. Feelings of rivalry with and resentment toward his pregnant partner

    c. Stressors

    d. Couvade

40. Monica Clark is 6 months pregnant and asks for advice about how to prepare her 3-year-old son Jared for the birth of a sibling. What suggestions might you give her?

*41. Pretend you are the head nurse in a prenatal clinic that provides care for women from a variety of ethnic backgrounds. You are responsible for orienting new nurses. Summarize three or four key points for the nurses to remember when caring for women from different cultures.

*These questions are addressed at the end of Part I.

Selected Answers

This section addresses the asterisked questions found in this chapter.

22. We are assuming you would take the time to find out if the comments bothered the woman and how she perceives her body image during pregnancy. In answer to her specific questions, you can point out that her "stomach-first walk" occurs because the weight and size of her growing uterus cause the center of gravity to change. To compensate, pregnant women tend to exaggerate the lumbar curve, which may result in backache. Because hormonal effects produce softening of the pelvic joints, the woman's walk assumes a more "waddling" appearance. This may be made more noticeable because many pregnant women also tend to walk with their feet farther apart to help maintain balance.

34. False results may occur with over-the-counter pregnancy tests if a test is performed too soon after a missed period. (Some tests require waiting until the ninth day; others may be done by the sixth day after a missed period.)

    False readings may also occur if a specimen other than the first of the day is used, because the first specimen contains the highest levels of hCG.

    Other factors that may contribute to a false reading include a dirty kit or a kit containing traces of soap or detergent, exposure of the sample to heat or sunlight, a sample that has stood longer than the specified time period, or movement of the test-tube sample during the timing period.

36. The effects of pregnancy on a woman's body image are greatly influenced by her feelings about her pregnancy and by cultural, physiologic, psychosocial, and interpersonal factors. Although the classic idea of the "glow of pregnancy"—a woman at her most lovely—has romantic appeal, it isn't necessarily true. When it does occur, it is most frequently seen in the second trimester when a woman has begun wearing maternity clothes. In the last weeks of pregnancy, a woman may feel constantly tired and misshapen and may, as a result, have a negative body image.

    You are on the right track if you recognized that a variety of factors influence body image and that, although there is no one correct answer, certain types of responses occur frequently.

37. Rubin identified the following psychologic tasks of the pregnant woman:

    a. Ensuring safe passage through pregnancy, labor, and birth. The woman's concern for herself and her unborn child leads her to select a care giver she trusts and to seek information about birth from classes, friends, and literature. She becomes more concerned about safety—both hers and her partner's.

    b. Seeking of acceptance of this child by others. The woman is concerned about her family's acceptance of the child, but her partner's reaction and acceptance are of primary importance to her successful completion of her developmental tasks. She also works to ensure the acceptance of the unborn child by other children in the family. The woman subtly alters her secondary network of friends as necessary to meet the demands of her pregnancy.

    c. Seeking of commitment and acceptance of self as mother to the infant—"binding-in." With quickening, the mother begins to develop bonds of attachment to the child and commits herself to the child's welfare.

    d. Learning to give of self on behalf of child. The woman begins to develop a capacity for self-denial and delayed personal gratification to meet the needs of another. Baby showers and gifts increase the mother's self-esteem while helping her accept the separateness and needs of her coming child.

38. We hope you would tell your friend that, even in the most desired pregnancy, feelings of ambivalence are normal. Role changes, physical changes, altered relationships, added financial responsibilities, and attitudes about parenting and values all affect a woman's, indeed a couple's, response to pregnancy.

41. It may be difficult initially for a nurse to recognize and accept cultural diversity. To do so the nurse needs to develop cultural sensitivity. The following points may help a nurse become more effective in caring for people from different cultures:

   a. We are all guilty of ethnocentrism occasionally. Ethnocentrism is the belief that one's own cultural beliefs and practices are the best ones. A nurse who finds herself or himself devaluing the practices of another culture should stop and consider that she or he may be demonstrating ethnocentrism.

   b. People have a tendency to project their own cultural responses onto people from another culture, and thus they assume that the person is acting from similar motives or values. Often this is not correct and leads to misunderstanding. For example, a nurse who highly values promptness may view a client's lateness as a personal insult when, in reality, the client is much less time-oriented and doesn't place the same value on promptness.

   c. Unless there is a clear health contraindication to a particular cultural practice, nurses should avoid interfering in a client's health practices. If the client's beliefs are potentially harmful, the nurse can try to persuade the woman to change. However, if the woman refuses to change, the nurse must accept the woman's right to make her own health choices.

   d. Before considering any intervention, the nurse should try to determine the impact of traditional practices on the planned intervention.

   e. Practices and beliefs vary not only from one culture to another but also *within* a culture. These variations are often related to social and economic factors such as class, income, and education.

   f. Nurses often find it helpful to begin developing cultural awareness by learning some of the basic beliefs and practices of minority cultures in their area.

If you included some of these ideas you are well on your way to developing cultural sensitivity. This is a challenging area for health care providers, and we hope you can become comfortable working with people from other cultures.

Part II Self-Assessment Guide

Do you know these abbreviations?

hCG   hPL

Add your own abbreviations or new words you have learned:

Can you answer these questions?

The following multiple-choice questions will help you assess your knowledge of the content of this chapter. Select the best answer for each of the questions and then refer to the end of Part II to check your answers.

1. The primary cause of uterine enlargement during pregnancy is the

   a. engorgement of preexisting vascular structures.

   b. formation of an additional layer of uterine musculature.

   c. hypertrophy of preexisting myometrial cells.

   d. increased number of myometrial cells.

2. During the first 10–12 weeks of pregnancy, the corpus luteum

   a. gradually regresses and becomes obliterated.

   b. secretes estrogen to maintain the pregnancy.

   c. secretes human chorionic gonadotropin to maintain the pregnancy.

   d. secretes progesterone to maintain the pregnancy.

3. During pregnancy, the increased number and activity of the endocervical glands are responsible for

   a. a marked softening of the cervix.

   b. a thinner, more watery mucosal discharge.

   c. the development of Chadwick's sign.

   d. the formation of the mucous plug.

4. The pseudoanemia of pregnancy is related to a decreased hematocrit, which is caused by

   a. a greater increase in plasma volume than in hemoglobin levels.

   b. decreased hemoglobin levels.

   c. a decrease in both plasma volume and hemoglobin levels.

   d. increased plasma volume without any concurrent increase in hemoglobin levels.

5. Which of the following hormones is similar to growth hormone in function and also contributes to the rise in blood glucose levels during pregnancy?

   a. Estrogen

   b. hCG

   c. hPL

   d. Progesterone

6. Constipation during pregnancy is usually the result of

   a. prolonged stomach emptying time and decreased intestinal motility.

   b. increased peristalsis and flatulence.

   c. increased cardiac work load resulting in delayed peristalsis.

   d. reflux of acidic gastric contents and hypochlorhydria.

7. Over-the-counter pregnancy tests determine the presence of hCG in the woman's

   a. blood.

   b. saliva.

   c. urine.

   d. vaginal secretions.

8. Which of the following changes in kidney functioning occurs during a normal pregnancy?

   a. Blood urea nitrogen values increase

   b. Glomerular filtration rate decreases

   c. Renal plasma flow increases

   d. Renal tubular reabsorption rate decreases

9. Which of the following is a probable sign of pregnancy?

    a. Amenorrhea

    b. Enlargement of the abdomen

    c. Nausea and vomiting

    d. Quickening

10. As her pregnancy progresses, Alana Lewis begins to see less of the women in her Young Businesswomen's Club and spends more time with two neighbors who have young children. Which of Rubin's psychologic tasks of pregnancy is she attempting to complete?

    a. Ensuring safe passage through pregnancy, labor, and birth

    b. Seeking of acceptance of this child by others

    c. Seeking of commitment and acceptance of self as mother to the infant

    d. Learning to give of self on behalf of child

Answers

1. c	2. d	3. d	4. a	5. c
6. a	7. c	8. c	9. b	10. b

Reference: Rubin R: *Maternal Identity and the Maternal Experience,* New York: Springer, 1984.

Nursing Assessment and Care of the Expectant Family

6

Introduction

The antepartal period is a time of great significance for both the expectant family and the unborn child. During this time, the family must adjust to the physical and psychologic changes occurring in the mother and must also come to terms with the impact a new baby will have on their own lives and roles. Nurses caring for the antepartal family must primarily consider the mother and her unborn child but cannot neglect the father, siblings, and others who form a significant part of the mother's support system.

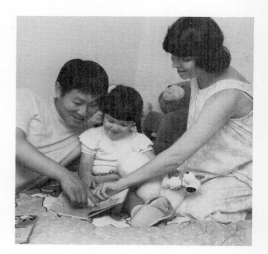

For the fetus, this is a time of unparalleled growth and development and also a time when his or her well-being is directly related to the mother's health, personal habits, and environment.

This chapter is designed to assist you in identifying common antepartal changes and health needs so that you may use this knowledge in assessing antepartal families and in planning, implementing, and evaluating their care. This chapter corresponds to Chapters 13, 14, 15, 16, and 17 in *Maternal-Newborn Nursing: A Family-Centered Approach,* 4th ed.

Part I Concepts, Critical Thinking, and Clinical Applications

1. Define the following terms, which are used when developing a woman's obstetric history:

   a. Gravida

   b. Primigravida

   c. Multigravida

   d. Para

e. Nullipara

f. Primipara

g. Multipara

h. Abortion

i. Stillbirth

j. Gestation

*2. Alexis Page is pregnant for the fourth time. She lost her first pregnancy at 12 weeks' gestation. She has two children at home. How would you record her obstetric history?

Gravida _____   Para _____   Ab _____   Living children _____

*3. a. Kerry Lawrence is pregnant for the third time. She delivered a stillborn infant at 36 weeks' gestation and has a three-year-old at home who was born at term. How would you record her obstetric history?

Gravida _____   Para _____   Ab _____   Living children _____

b. A more detailed approach can also be used. In this approach, the meaning of *gravida* remains unchanged while *para* changes slightly to focus on the number of infants born. Use the acronym *TPAL* to remember *T*erm, *P*reterm *A*bortions, *L*iving children. Using this method, how would you record Kerry's obstetric history?

Gravida _____   Para __ __ __ __

*These questions are addressed at the end of Part I.

*4.   The following questionnaire is similar to many that are used when a woman initially seeks antepartal care. With a friend or family member acting as the client and you as the prenatal nurse, obtain the necessary information. (Note: This questionnaire focuses primarily on factors related to pregnancy and is not a complete history of all body systems.)

Name: _____ Age: _____ Race: _____

Address: _____ Phone: _____

Educational level: _____ Occupation: _____

Marital status: _____ Religious preference (optional) _____

Have any members of your family had the following? If so, who?

_____ Diabetes _____

_____ Cardiovascular disease _____

_____ High blood pressure _____

_____ Breast cancer _____

_____ Other types of cancer _____

_____ Multiple pregnancies _____

_____ Preeclampsia-eclampsia (pregnancy-induced hypertension) _____

_____ Congenital anomalies _____

How old were you when your menstrual periods started? _____

How often do they occur? _____

How long do they last? _____

Do you have any discomfort with your periods? _____ If so, how severe is it? _____

What is the date of the first day of your last normal menstrual period? _____

Have you had any bleeding or spotting since your last normal menstrual period? _____

Have you had any of the following diseases?

_____ Chickenpox	_____ Asthma
_____ Mumps	_____ High blood pressure
_____ Three-day measles (rubella)	_____ Heart disease
_____ Two-week measles (rubeola)	_____ Respiratory disease
_____ Kidney disease	_____ Diabetes
_____ Frequent bladder infections	_____ Allergies
_____ Thyroid problems	_____ Sexually transmitted infection
_____ Anemia	_____ Other

(If the woman answers *yes* to any of the above, include pertinent information in this space.)

*These questions are addressed at the end of Part I.

Have you been on birth control pills? _____ If yes, when did you stop taking them? _____

Were you using any other method of contraception? _____ If so, what method? _____

How many previous pregnancies have you had? _____

Have you had any miscarriages or abortions? _____ If yes, how many? _____

How many living children do you have? _____

Have you had any stillbirths? _____ If yes, how many? _____

Gravida _____ Para _____ Ab _____

Previous children:

Date of birth	Sex	Birthweight	Preterm or full term
1.			
2.			
3.			
4.			
5.			

Did any previous children have problems immediately after birth? _____ If yes, what occurred?

Have you had any problems with previous pregnancies? _____ If yes, what occurred?

Have you had any problems with previous labors and/or births? _____ If yes, what occurred?

Have you had any problems with previous postpartal periods? _____ If yes, what occurred?

Are you presently taking any prescription or nonprescription drugs? _____ If yes, please list them.

1.   3.

2.   4.

Do you smoke? _____ Number of cigarettes per day: _____

How much of the following do you drink per day?

1. Coffee

2. Tea

3. Colas

4. Alcoholic beverages

What is your present weight? _____ What is your usual prepregnant weight? _____

Nursing assessment of available psychosocial data (to be completed by nurse using information obtained from the patient or other sources):**

Brief description of available support persons (include marital status and information about the father of the child, such as age, occupation, involvement in the pregnancy):

Client feelings about the pregnancy:

Plans for adapting to the pregnancy:

Any cultural or religious practices that might influence the client's care or that of her child:

**This should be a brief summary of your impression of the woman, her ability to cope with her pregnancy, plans she has made, and available support systems.

5. The following blood tests are frequently done during the initial physical exam. List the normal findings and the rationale for each.

Test	Normal Findings	Rationale
Serology		
Hematocrit		
Hemoglobin		
White blood cells (WBC)		
ABO and Rh typing		
Rubella titer		

6. A urinalysis and urine culture and sensitivity are also done. What types of abnormal findings are possible and what is their significance?

7. During the prenatal assessment, the woman is screened for risk factors. What are risk factors?

_____

_____

_____

8. Give three examples of factors that increase a woman's risk:

a.

b.

c.

The procedure for a complete physical examination may be reviewed in textbooks on physical assessment. This workbook focuses on those aspects of the physical examination that are directly related to assessment of the pregnancy.

*9. Allison Scott, gravida 1 para 0 ab 0, is scheduled for her first obstetric examination. Identify three areas of focus in this examination.

a.

b.

c.

10. During her examination, the nurse-practitioner (or physician) measures Allison's fundal height. How is this measured?

11. a. What information does fundal height provide about the pregnancy?

b. Where would you expect to find the fundus at 12 weeks' gestation? _____

At 20 weeks'? _____

12. Allison asks you when the baby's heartbeat will be heard. When is the fetal heartbeat usually detected?

a. With a fetoscope: _____

b. With a Doppler: _____

13. To complete a pelvic examination, Allison is placed in the _____ position.

*14. Identify the three basic parts of every initial pelvic examination.

a.

b.

c.

*These questions are addressed at the end of Part I.

15. Adequacy of the maternal pelvic diameters is usually determined prenatally. Label the pelvic diameters depicted in Figure 6–1. Complete the accompanying chart.

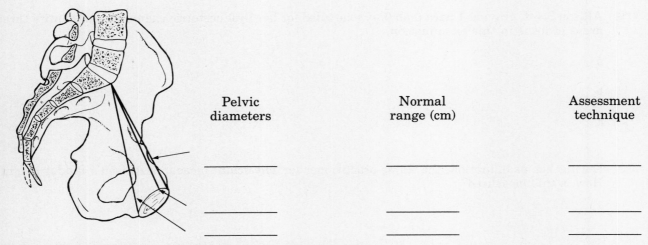

Pelvic diameters	Normal range (cm)	Assessment technique
_____	_____	_____
_____	_____	_____
_____	_____	_____

Figure 6–1 Anteroposterior diameters of the pelvic inlet.

*16. If you noted on a prenatal record that a woman had a diagonal conjugate of 9.0 cm, what possible problems might you predict for her labor? What problems might be associated with converging side walls? With incurving coccyx?

17. State Nägele's rule. _____

_____

How accurate is it?

*18. Allison began her last normal menstrual period on March 22 of this year. Using Nägele's rule, calculate her expected date of birth (EDB).

19. What is the recommended frequency of prenatal visits for a normal prenatal client?

20. Identify the factors that you would consider part of your initial psychologic assessment of an antepartal family.

21. What behaviors might indicate psychologic problems in relation to the pregnancy?

22. During Allison's initial prenatal visit, you discuss the danger signals of pregnancy with her. Identify at least eight danger signals and explain the possible significance of each.

Danger Signal	Significance
a.	
b.	
c.	
d.	
e.	
f.	
g.	
h.	

23. What will you instruct Allison to do if she should experience any of the danger signals?

24. The following chart lists discomforts that commonly occur during pregnancy. For each discomfort, briefly describe the cause and possible interventions for alleviating it.

Discomfort	Time of Occurrence	Cause	Method of Alleviation
Nausea/vomiting			
Nasal stuffiness and epistaxis			
Urinary frequency			
Breast tenderness			
Ptyalism			
Increased vaginal discharge			
Heartburn			
Ankle edema			
Varicose veins			
Hemorrhoids			
Flatulence			
Constipation			
Backache			
Leg cramps			
Faintness			
Shortness of breath			
Difficulty sleeping			
Round ligament pain			
Carpal tunnel syndrome			

The following action sequence is designed to help you think through basic clinical problems. We've answered portions of it at the end of Part I.

*25. **Action Sequence**
Kerry Lynd, G1 P0, is 12 weeks pregnant when she comes for her second prenatal visit. She tells you that her main problem is noticeable fatigue. She states, "Sometimes I'm so tired by the end of the day that I can hardly make it home to cook supper. I can't tell you how many meals Larry has cooked lately because I don't have the energy to do it. Is something wrong with me?"

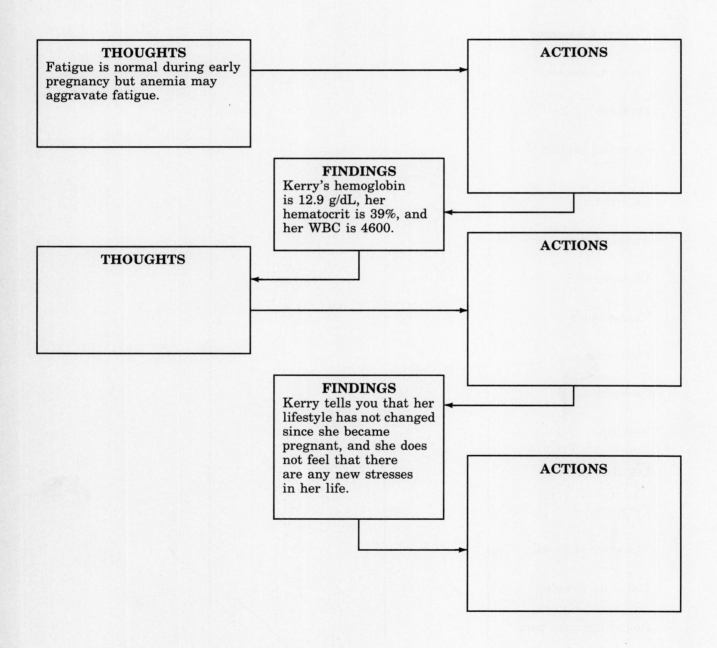

26. Allison Scott is interested in breast-feeding her baby and asks if there is anything she should do during pregnancy to prepare her breasts. What advice would you give her?

27. Allison asks about the types of physical activity she can engage in during pregnancy. What guidelines would you suggest she follow when engaging in sports and physical activities?

28. In counseling pregnant women about their activities, what information would you provide about the following?

   a. Bathing

   b. Employment

   c. Travel

   d. Appropriate prenatal exercises

   e. Sexual activities

   f. Dental care

   g. Medications

   h. Smoking

   i. Alcohol

   j. Caffeine

   k. Social drugs

*29. Kathy Wilson is 7 months pregnant with her first child. She tells you that she and her partner, Chuck, still find sexual intercourse very satisfying, although recently they have found it more comfortable to make love if Kathy assumes the superior position. Kathy says that she and Chuck recently talked about making love during the last weeks of pregnancy. They wondered if it was "OK" or if it posed a threat for Kathy or the baby. After assessing Kathy's concerns, formulate an appropriate nursing diagnosis.

Based on your nursing diagnosis, briefly outline a plan to meet Kathy's needs.

Age-Related Considerations

30. Identify at least six reasons why an adolescent might become pregnant.

a.

b.

c.

d.

e.

f.

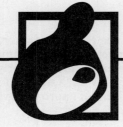

It's Your Turn

Think about any pregnant adolescents you have cared for as a nursing student or have known. Compare their reactions to being pregnant to those of more mature pregnant women. How are they similar? Different?

_____

_____

_____

_____

_____

_____

_____

_____

_____

_____

_____

_____

_____

_____

_____

_____

_____

_____

_____

*31. Pretend you are responsible for developing a prenatal clinic for adolescent girls. What factors about the adolescent and her development would you consider in planning your approach? Identify some specific techniques or services you would like to have available for the adolescent.

32. Identify some of the special concerns of the older expectant couple.

Maternal Nutrition

33. Diana Cooper, a 22-year-old primipara, 2 months pregnant, is discussing nutrition with you. She is of normal weight and is very concerned about avoiding excessive weight gain. What pattern of weight gain would you recommend for her?

34. To achieve this weight gain, she should increase her daily intake by _____ kcal.

_____

*These questions are addressed at the end of Part I.

35. What recommendations might you give Diana about achieving this increase in a nutritionally sound way?

36. What are the functions of the following categories of nutrients?

    a. Protein

    b. Carbohydrates

    c. Fat

37. For each of the following vitamins or minerals, briefly describe its functions and identify some common food sources:

Vitamin/Mineral	Function	Sources
Vitamin A		
Vitamin D		
Vitamin E		
Vitamin K		

Vitamin/Mineral	Function	Sources
Vitamin C		
Thiamine (B$_1$)		
Riboflavin (B$_2$)		
Niacin		
Folic acid		
Pantothenic acid		
Pyridoxin (B$_6$)		
Cobalamin (B$_{12}$)		

Vitamin/Mineral	Function	Sources
Calcium		
Phosphorus		
Iodine		
Sodium		
Zinc		
Magnesium		
Iron		

*38. Tina Nelson is a true vegetarian and will not eat any food from animal sources, including milk and eggs. What foods might she use to meet her protein and calcium requirements during pregnancy?

*39. The following is a 24-hour food diary for a 26-year-old pregnant woman of normal weight. Analyze its adequacy with regard to the basic food groups.

Breakfast
    3/4 oz dry cereal
    1/2 cup low-fat milk
    4 oz orange juice

Lunch:
    Sandwich made with 2 slices whole wheat bread, 2 oz chicken breast, lettuce, mayonnaise
    8 oz milk
    1 small chocolate bar

Dinner:
    6 oz flounder
    tossed salad with dressing
    1/2 cup rice
    1 piece of cake

Snack:
    1 1/2 cup vanilla ice cream

Analysis:

Dairy products:

Meat group:

Grains:

Fruits and vegetables:

---

*These questions are addressed at the end of Part I.

40. Define pica.

41. How might the nurse identify the woman who practices pica?

42. What special factors should be considered in helping pregnant adolescents meet their nutritional needs?

*43. Your client, Elena Montoya, of normal weight initially, is now 18 weeks pregnant. She has gained 32 pounds to date. Her history and physical examination are otherwise normal. You formulate the nursing diagnosis "Altered nutrition: More than body requirements related to excessive caloric intake." Your interventions include discussions about the importance of appropriate weight gain and classes in meal planning and preparation with the nutritionist, who is sensitive to the importance of respecting cultural preferences about food. What approaches might you use to evaluate the effectiveness of your nursing care plan?

Preparation for Childbirth

44. During pregnancy, the expectant family begins to plan for their childbirth experience. Identify at least six issues a family should consider in their decision making.

    a.

    b.

    c.

    d.

    e.

    f.

45. Many types of prenatal classes are available for expectant women/couples. Identify three and list the main goals of each.

46. Compare the Lamaze method of childbirth preparation to a method commonly used in your area with regard to philosophy and basic approaches.

Selected Answers

This section addresses the asterisked questions found in this chapter.

2. Alexis is a gravida 4 para 2 ab 1 living children 2.

3. a. Kerry is a gravida 3 para 2 ab 0 living children 1. If you recorded this differently, was it because you forgot that a stillborn infant would be considered viable at 36 weeks and would therefore count as a para?

   b. Using the detailed approach, Kerry would be a gravida 3 para 1101. Kerry's stillborn infant would be considered a preterm delivery.

4. Taking an obstetric health history should help you focus on the information that is pertinent to high-quality maternity care. You should be able to identify a reason for each of the questions asked. You should also be able to identify information that may place a client in the high-risk category. In addition to such obvious problems as preexisting medical conditions, think about maternal age, weight, occupation, and previous obstetric history; family history of disorders; marital status and support system; smoking and alcohol consumption; and so on. Once you begin to recognize risk factors, you will be better able to plan for appropriate antepartal care.

9. The initial obstetric examination focuses on

   a. inspection, auscultation, and palpation of the abdomen.

   b. determination of the adequacy of the pelvis.

   c. vaginal examination.

14. The initial pelvic examination should include

   a. a Pap smear and any other pertinent cultures or smears.

   b. visual inspection of the external genitalia, vagina, and cervix.

   c. a bimanual examination.

16. A diagonal conjugate of 9.0 cm indicates a severely diminished pelvic inlet. In this case, if labor were to occur, the fetal head would probably not be able to enter the pelvic outlet. In spite of uterine contractions, the fetal head would not engage, and the presenting part would probably be described as ballotable, or floating. When a measurement such as this is discovered during the prenatal course, the woman is counseled regarding the need for cesarean birth.

   Problems associated with converging side walls refer to a condition in which the sides of the midpelvis are farther apart at the top than at the bottom. The resulting shape is similar to that of a funnel. In this case, the fetal head may engage but fetal descent is very slow or not possible. When the woman is in labor, there will be very slow fetal descent, which is indicated by no change or minimal change in station. The fetal head may develop a caput succedaneum due to prolonged pressure on the fetal scalp.

   An incurving coccyx may hinder the descent of the fetal head in the later part of the first stage of labor. In some instances, the inward curve is great enough to completely block passage of the fetus, and a cesarean is done.

18. Allison's EDB would be December 29 ($\pm$ 2 weeks). If you count back February, January, December, it is easy to identify the month. If you set it up as a problem, it is a little more difficult:

March 22 becomes	3 — 21
Subtract 3 months	−3
	0 — 22
Add 7 days	+ 7
EDB	0 — 29

If you remember that January is always the first month, then an answer of "0" becomes December, an answer of "minus 1" would be November, and "minus 2" would be October.

25. *Actions:* In most clinics and offices, laboratory tests are completed at the initial prenatal visit. Thus you could quickly refer to the results of the hemoglobin and hematocrit to determine if Kerry is anemic.

Thoughts: Kerry's lab values are within normal limits, so you know she is not anemic. It is tempting at this point to simply assume the fatigue is normal because it is so common among pregnant women. However, this assumption might lead you to miss factors in Kerry's life that are contributing to the problem—extra stress at work, the stress of helping a family member with a sick child, or frequent awakenings at night for trips to the bathroom.

Actions: An appropriate action might be to provide reassurance while pursuing the matter. You might say, for example, "Many women feel tired during the early months of pregnancy, but sometimes factors or events in the woman's life can add to the fatigue. Is there anything happening in your life that you feel might be contributing to the fatigue?"

Actions: Kerry's indication that her life-style is unchanged suggests that the fatigue is a normal part of her pregnancy. At this point you can begin working with her to plan ways she can get more rest during the day.

29. A possible nursing diagnosis would be "Knowledge deficit related to guidelines for sexual activity during the third trimester." Perhaps you chose "Sexual dysfunction related to lack of knowledge." It is tempting because the problem concerns sexual activity, and some people would support this diagnosis. However, because their sexual activity is satisfying to both and they have adapted their practices in light of the pregnancy, they do not meet the definition of a dysfunction. They are simply seeking information.

31. This question gives you a lot of room to plan creatively. Obviously, there is no one right answer. We hope that in planning your clinic you keep in mind that the early adolescent is often quite different in needs and interaction from the late adolescent. Although the older adolescent can often think abstractly, many adolescents are very concrete thinkers and tend to be present-oriented and egocentric. Thus it is helpful to use audiovisual aids and provide "hands-on" learning experiences. Activities have more meaning if the adolescent sees them as having a specific value for her.

In planning we hope you emphasize a multidisciplinary approach that also includes the father of the child and the parents of the adolescent mother and father (if the adolescents wish them to be involved). This leads to the question of choice: It is important to give these adolescents choices and to help them learn to make appropriate decisions. Thus some guidance may be beneficial, but too much may keep them from learning how to make choices and decisions.

Finally, we hope you give some thought to the atmosphere of your clinic: Is it open, nonjudgmental, and supportive? Do the adolescents feel free to ask questions and express fears? Does it feel safe and free of coercion?

38. Pregnant vegetarians often use soybean products such as soybean milk, tofu, and soy protein isolates as a source of protein. Other sources include nuts and lentils. Possible additional sources of calcium include turnip greens, white beans, and almonds.

39. This woman's diet had 4 servings of grain products. This is adequate. She had 4 servings of protein, which is more than adequate. However, since she only had 2 1/2 servings of dairy products (recommended is 4) and 3 fruits or vegetables (4–6 are recommended), her diet is deficient in these areas.

43. Evaluation is, indeed, an important part of the nursing process. Choose evaluation methods that are simple, easily implemented, and logical. You may have Elena come in weekly to be weighed, for example, and may also ask her to keep a food diary for a week or so. You may also schedule follow-up visits with the nutritionist, who can gently quiz Elena about her diet and her understanding of good nutrition. Perhaps you have thought of other activities as well.

Part II Self-Assessment Guide

Do you know these abbreviations?

DFMR	EDB
EDC	EDD
FAD	G
P	RDA

Add your own abbreviations or new words you have learned:

Can you answer these questions?

The following multiple-choice questions will help you assess your knowledge of the content of this chapter. Select the best answer for each of the questions and then refer to the end of Part II to check your answers.

1. Molly Higgins is pregnant again. She has two living children at home. A third child died of birth defects at 4 days of age. She has never had an abortion. Which of the following most accurately describes her now?
   a. Gravida 3 para 2 ab O
   b. Gravida 3 para 3 ab O
   c. Gravida 4 para 2 ab 1
   d. Gravida 4 para 3 ab O

2. Molly has a hemoglobin of 13 gm/dL and a hematocrit of 41%. Which of the following statements about these values is most accurate?
   a. Both are within normal limits.
   b. Hemoglobin is normal; hematocrit indicates a physiologic anemia.
   c. Hemoglobin indicates an iron deficiency anemia; hematocrit is normal.
   d. Hemoglobin and hematocrit are elevated and indicate polycythemia.

3. Molly began her last normal menstrual period on November 19. Her estimated date of birth (EDB) is
   a. August 12.
   b. August 26.
   c. September 16.
   d. September 19.

4. Which of the common discomforts of pregnancy listed below generally have their initial onset during the first half of pregnancy?
   a. Backache
   b. Dyspnea
   c. Fatigue
   d. Varicose veins

5. Your friend is in her early months of pregnancy and complains about morning sickness. Which of the following recommendations might you make to her?
   a. Nothing will alleviate it, and you must do your best to accept it.
   b. Eat a dry carbohydrate, such as crackers, before arising.
   c. Take large quantities of fluids with meals.
   d. Eat three meals per day and avoid eating between meals.

6. A woman experiencing constipation during pregnancy should be advised to increase her dietary intake of
   a. dairy products.
   b. fresh fruits and vegetables.
   c. poultry and seafood.
   d. refined flour products.

7. Which of the following symptoms should a woman be instructed to report to her health care provider immediately?
   a. Ankle edema
   b. Heartburn
   c. Urinary frequency
   d. Vaginal bleeding

8. A child born to a woman over age 35 has an increased risk of
   a. Down syndrome.
   b. cleft palate.
   c. cystic fibrosis.
   d. meningomyelocele.

9. Which of the following menus would provide the highest amounts of protein, iron, and vitamin C?
   a. 4 oz beef, 1/2 c lima beans, a glass of skim milk, and 3/4 c strawberries
   b. 3 oz chicken, 1/2 c corn, a lettuce salad, and a small banana
   c. 1 c macaroni, 3/4 c peas, a glass of whole milk, and a medium pear
   d. A scrambled egg, a hash-browned potato, half a glass of buttermilk, and a large nectarine

10. For the pregnant adolescent, the most common medical complication is
    a. gestational diabetes mellitus.
    b. herpes simplex.
    c. pregnancy-induced hypertension.
    d. pyelonephritis.

Answers

1. d	2. a	3. b	4. c	5. b
6. b	7. d	8. a	9. a	10. c

Pregnancy at Risk

Introduction

An at-risk pregnancy is one in which certain factors or groups of factors increase the possibility of morbidity or even mortality for the mother and/or fetus (or neonate).

This chapter delineates the personal, social, cultural, and environmental factors that might increase the risk. Preexisting conditions, such as maternal heart disease, are then explored, followed by disorders that develop during pregnancy. The final portion of the chapter discusses the infectious processes that may pose a significant threat to maternal, fetal, or neonatal well-being. The chapter corresponds to Chapters 18 and 19 in *Maternal-Newborn Nursing: A Family-Centered Approach,* 4th ed.

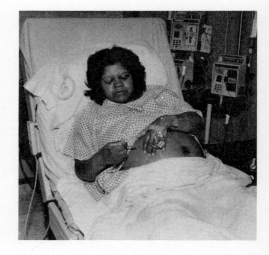

Part I Concepts, Critical Thinking, and Clinical Applications

Pregestational Problems

1. Identify three changes that normally occur in the cardiovascular system during pregnancy.

   a.

   b.

   c.

2. The New York Heart Association classification of functional capacity is used to assess the severity of cardiac disease. For each of the classes, state the expected physical activity level.

   a. Class I

   b. Class II

   c. Class III

   d. Class IV

3. Sandy Carson is a 24-year-old woman who had rheumatic fever as a child and is now considered a class II cardiac client. List five signs and symptoms that would lead you to suspect cardiac decompensation in Sandy.

   a.

   b.

   c.

   d.

   e.

4. During the antepartal period, what information would you give Sandy about the following?

   a. Nutrition

   b. Rest

   c. Protection from infection

   d. Activity level and restrictions

   e. Frequency of prenatal visits

5. In addition to iron and vitamin supplements, Sandy is started on penicillin prophylaxis. Why is this done?

*6. In the absence of complications, what is the method of choice by which Sandy would give birth?

Diabetes Mellitus and Pregnancy

7. Define the following as they are used in the classification of diabetes mellitus developed by the National Diabetes Data Group:

a. Diabetes mellitus

   Type I, insulin dependent (IDDM)

   Type II, noninsulin dependent (NIDDM)

   Secondary diabetes

b. Impaired glucose tolerance (IGT)

c. Gestational diabetes (GDM)

8. Pregnancy has been described as having a diabetogenic effect.

a. Define the diabetogenic effect of pregnancy.

b. Identify three physiologic factors that contribute to the diabetogenic effect of pregnancy.

   i.

   ii.

   iii.

*These questions are addressed at the end of Part I.

9. Identify five maternal and/or fetal complications that may occur during pregnancy as a result of diabetes mellitus.

   a.

   b.

   c.

   d.

   e.

*10. Belle Arthur, a 29-year-old G2 P1, was diagnosed as having diabetes mellitus a year ago. Her diabetes was controlled with low doses of insulin. When her pregnancy was diagnosed at 7 weeks gestation, her glycosylated hemoglobin was 6.4% and her fasting blood glucose (FBG) was 98 mg/dL. Belle missed her last two prenatal visits but states that she carefully followed her diet and insulin dosage schedule. Today's FBG is 102 mg/dL and her glycosylated hemoglobin is 7.0%. Did Ms Arthur maintain effective control?_____ Explain your answer.

*11. You ask Ms Arthur why she missed her last two appointments. She tells you that she depends on a neighbor for a ride, and her neighbor's car was broken. Because of the location of her home, she would have to transfer twice if she took a bus. Based on this data, what nursing diagnosis might you formulate?

---

*These questions are addressed at the end of Part I.

*12. You ask Ms Arthur if she can think of anything that would make it easier for her to keep her appointments. She states, "There is a satellite clinic really close to my house, but they won't see me because they say I'm high risk." You know that Belle's physician works at that clinic one day a week. You explain the situation and ask if she would be willing to see Belle there. The physician agrees, and Belle is delighted with the change. Evaluate the effectiveness of your intervention.

13. In caring for a pregnant woman with diabetes mellitus, what general information would you give her about the following areas of concern?

   a. Dietary regulation

   b. Home glucose monitoring

   c. Insulin requirements

   d. Exercise

   e. Symptoms of hypoglycemia

   f. Frequency of prenatal visits

*14. A friend of yours is diagnosed as having gestational diabetes. She tells you that her grandmother takes tolbutamide (Orinase) for her diabetes and asks why she can't simply take tolbutamide too. What would you tell her?

---

*These questions are addressed at the end of Part I.

15. Your friend also asks why infants of diabetic mothers are often large at birth. How would you explain this phenomenon?

16. List three tests that might be performed to assess fetal status in a pregnant woman with diabetes.

    a.

    b.

    c.

17. Identify signs of acquired immunodeficiency syndrome (AIDS) that may occur in infants born to human immunodeficiency virus (HIV)–positive women.

18. List four groups of women who should be screened for a positive HIV.

    a.

    b.

    c.

    d.

19. Briefly discuss guidelines for counseling for women who test HIV–positive.

20. Summarize the Centers for Disease Control (CDC) guidelines (universal precautions) for preventing the transmission of AIDS.

21. Identify the risks to a fetus/neonate of a woman who abuses the following:

    a. Alcohol

    b. Cocaine

    c. Marijuana

    d. Heroin

Gestational Onset Problems

22. Define *hyperemesis gravidarum.*

23. Identify the goals of therapy in treating a woman hospitalized with hyperemesis gravidarum.

Bleeding Disorders

Bleeding at any time during pregnancy is considered a potential problem and requires evaluation. Spontaneous abortion (miscarriage) is the major bleeding disorder associated with the first and second trimesters of pregnancy.

24. Match the terms below with the correct definitions:

_____ Threatened abortion   a. Loss of three or more successive pregnancies

_____ Imminent abortion   b. Abortion characterized by vaginal bleeding and cramping but a closed cervical os

_____ Complete abortion   c. Abortion in which the fetus dies in utero but is not expelled

_____ Incomplete abortion   d. Abortion in which all the products of conception are expelled

_____ Missed abortion   e. Abortion characterized by bleeding, cramping, and dilatation of the cervical os

_____ Habitual abortion   f. Abortion in which a portion of the products of conception is retained

25. Alys Roberts, a 22-year-old gravida 1 para 0, 11 weeks pregnant, was admitted to the hospital with moderate vaginal bleeding and some abdominal cramping. Vaginal examination reveals that the cervix is dilated 2 cm. She is diagnosed as having an imminent abortion. Identify four nursing interventions that are indicated in caring for Alys.

a.

b.

c.

d.

26. Alys is placed on bedrest with intravenous fluids and that evening passes some of the products of conception. The following morning she has a dilation and curettage (D & C). Why is this done?

27. Alys husband asks you why abortions occur. Identify four causes of spontaneous abortion.

    a.

    b.

    c.

    d.

28. The most common cause of second-trimester abortion is incompetent cervix. Identify two factors that may contribute to incompetent cervix.

    a.

    b.

29. A surgical procedure used to treat incompetent cervix so that a woman may successfully carry a pregnancy to term is _____ .

30. Define *ectopic pregnancy*.

31. The most common implantation site in an ectopic pregnancy is the _____ .

32. Lindsay Albertson is seen at your office with a possible ectopic pregnancy. She tells you that she has two friends who have had ectopic pregnancies and asks you if they are becoming more common. How would you respond?

33. Ectopic pregnancy is often difficult to diagnose because its symptoms are similar to those of abdominal conditions. Identify at least five signs or symptoms of ectopic pregnancy and briefly explain why each occurs.

Sign or Symptom	Physiologic Rationale for Occurrence
a.	
b.	
c.	
d.	
e.	

34. Lindsay asks you how ectopic pregnancy is diagnosed. How would you respond?

35. Lucy Harris is admitted with a diagnosis of gestational trophoblastic disease. Define *gestational trophoblastic disease.*

36. What signs and symptoms might Lucy have exhibited that would lead to this diagnosis?

a.

b.

c.

d.

e.

*37. Following successful removal of the mole, Ms Harris is advised to avoid pregnancy for a year and to return for periodic measurement of human chorionic gonadotropin (hCG) levels. What is the rationale for this advice?

Preterm Labor

38. Sarah Smythe is 36 years old and is a gravida 4. She has two children at home; one of them was born at 35 weeks' gestation. Sarah had one spontaneous abortion. She smokes 10 cigarettes a day and has an occasional glass of wine. Sarah has a history of pyelonephritis. She has been working for the past 2 years in a factory. Her job requires that she stand in one place along a conveyor belt and inspect parts as they pass by. Sarah had a brief episode of vaginal bleeding at 14 weeks' gestation, which lasted 2 days. Since then, the pregnancy has gone well; however, she has noted more contractions lately.

*a. Circle all of Mrs Smythe's risk factors for preterm labor.

*b. Mrs Smythe asks you what she should look for this time. Identify important information to include in your answer.

*These questions are addressed at the end of Part I.

*c. Mrs Smythe receives your information in a serious, thoughtful manner. At the end of your conversation, she says "But how do I know if it's a real contraction?" What assessment techniques will you teach her?

d. Mrs Smythe tells you that even though one of her babies was premature, she still does not understand why the baby had so many problems. "He looked all right. He was just small." Write out your explanation of the special problems that preterm babies have.

*39. There are many signs and symptoms associated with preterm labor. When any of the signs and symptoms of preterm labor are present, it is important for the woman to call her health care provider and be evaluated in a health care birth setting. Place an "X" beside all factors in the following list that would need further evaluation:

_____ nausea   _____ headache (mild) relieved by resting and cool cloth to forehead

_____ diarrhea   _____ backache

_____ thirst   _____ unusual tiredness

_____ cramps in legs   _____ increased appetite

40. Mrs Smythe is admitted in preterm labor at 30 weeks' gestation and is started on intravenous (IV) ritodrine (Yutopar).

a. How does this drug work?

b. Why is the drug contraindicated in women with

(1) pregnancy-induced hypertension?

(2) diabetes mellitus?

(3) cardiac disease?

*c. The IV fluid Sarah is receiving contains 150 mg ritodrine in 500 mL of IV fluid, and the resulting dilution is 0.3 mg/mL. The initial dose is 0.1 mg/min, which is equal to 20 mL/hr on an adult infusion pump. To administer the maximum dosage of 0.35 mg/min, the infusion pump will be set at _____ mL/hr.

d. Why may the obstetrician order an electrocardiogram and serum potassium for the woman receiving ritodrine intravenously?

e. When the ritodrine is being increased, careful nursing assessments are important. For each of the following, identify the most important nursing assessments and rationale:

	Assessment	Rationale
Maternal pulse	Check pulse every 15 minutes to detect tachycardia	Pulse above 140 alters perfusion
Maternal B/P		
Maternal lab values		
Blood glucose		
Potassium		
Maternal lungs		
Fetal heart rate		

f. Sometimes we discuss complications without reviewing normal assessments presented in classes other than childbearing classes. If you need a review, complete the following:

Fluid intake for an adult is _____ mL per 24 hours. Normal output is _____ mL per hour and _____ mL per 24 hours.

Normal vital signs are: B/P ____/____ ; P _____ ; R _____ .

Label pictorial representations of breath sounds.

$\bigwedge$ _____ $\bigwedge$ _____ $\bigwedge$ _____

Normal lab value for serum potassium is _____ .

Normal lab value for blood glucose is _____ .

41. Some women who are receiving a maintenance dose of ritodrine may also be given betamethasone.

a. The usual dose and route are _____ .

b. It is important for the oral ritodrine to be taken on time. How would you explain this to a woman so that she thoroughly understands the reasons for it?

*c. List the most important information to include in your discharge teaching for the woman receiving oral ritodrine.

42. Identify two nursing diagnoses you think are important for a woman in preterm labor. Include your supporting data for the nursing diagnoses.

*These questions are addressed at the end of Part I.

*43. The following situation has been included to challenge your critical thinking. Read the situation and then answer the question "yes" or "no."

  a. Mrs Quick is admitted to the birthing unit, and you will be responsible for her care. She is a G 4, P 3, ab 0, living children 3, term birth 1, preterm births 2. She is 34 weeks' gestation and is having contractions every 3 minutes of 40 seconds duration. She states that her membranes have been ruptured since yesterday at noon (23 hours ago). In your initial assessments, you find FHR 140, T 99.2, P 92, R 18, cervical dilatation 5 cm, and Nitrazine positive.

_____ **Is Mrs Quick a candidate for treatment to stop labor?** _____
⇓   ⇓

Yes (Why? _____)   No (Why not? _____)

Identify the therapy you would expect   Identify your most pressing nursing goal.
to be initiated.

  b. Mrs Allen is admitted in preterm labor at 32 weeks' gestation. In the first few minutes of care, many nursing actions are needed. Rank the nursing actions in order of priority. Place NA (not applicable) by those actions that could be deleted at this time.

_____ Apply electronic monitor to determine contraction frequency and duration and FHR

_____ Assess maternal B/P, TPR

_____ Complete all sections of the admission form

_____ Do a sterile vaginal examination to determine dilatation, effacement, fetal station, presentation, and position

_____ Use Nitrazine to test for ruptured membranes

_____ Weigh Mrs Allen

_____ Listen to breath sounds

  c. Mrs Golden is admitted in preterm labor and ritodrine IV therapy is to be initiated STAT. Rank the following nursing actions in order of priority. Place NA by those that could and/or should be deleted at this time.

_____ Assess uterine contraction frequency, duration, and intensity by palpation

_____ Obtain maternal vital signs (B/P, TPR) for a baseline

_____ Prepare ritodrine infusion

_____ Apply an electronic fetal monitor (EFM)

_____

*These questions are addressed at the end of Part I.

Pregnancy-Induced Hypertension (PIH)

The following action sequence is designed to help you think through basic clinical problems. We've answered portions of it at the end of Part I.

*44. **Action Sequence**
You work as a professional nurse in a private obstetrician's office. Rita George, G1 P0, 37 weeks pregnant, is in for her weekly prenatal appointment. When you weigh her you note that she has gained 2 3/4 lb since last week. Her pregnancy to date has been completely normal. You know that the average weight gain in the last trimester is about 1 lb/week. A large weight gain often indicates that fluid is being retained. You know that this is an early sign of preeclampsia.

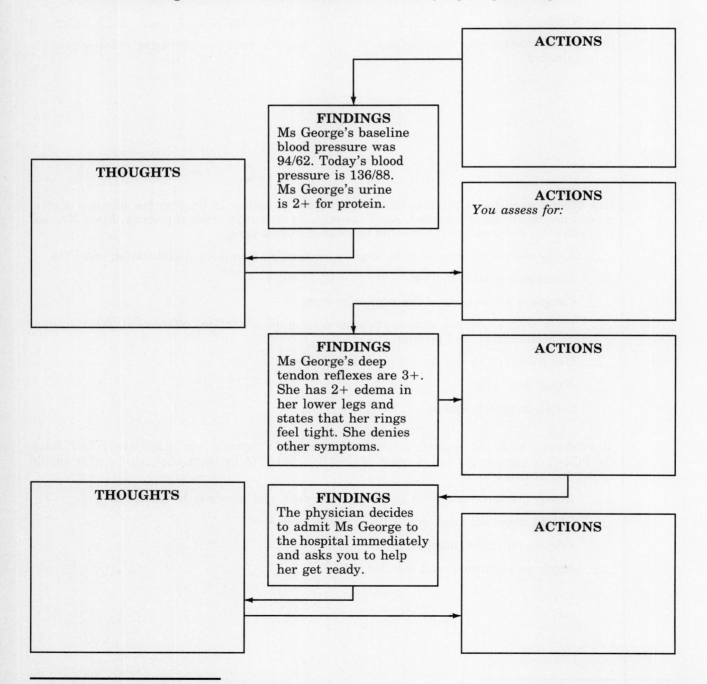

ACTIONS

FINDINGS
Ms George's baseline blood pressure was 94/62. Today's blood pressure is 136/88. Ms George's urine is 2+ for protein.

THOUGHTS

ACTIONS
You assess for:

FINDINGS
Ms George's deep tendon reflexes are 3+. She has 2+ edema in her lower legs and states that her rings feel tight. She denies other symptoms.

ACTIONS

THOUGHTS

FINDINGS
The physician decides to admit Ms George to the hospital immediately and asks you to help her get ready.

ACTIONS

---

*These questions are addressed at the end of Part I.

45. On the following chart, compare the signs and symptoms of mild preeclampsia and severe preeclampsia (pregnancy-induced hypertension):

Sign	Mild Preeclampsia	Severe Preeclampsia
Blood pressure		
Weight gain		
Edema		
Proteinuria		
Hyperreflexia		
Headache		
Epigastric pain		
Visual disturbances		

46. What additional symptom characterizes a woman as having eclampsia rather than severe preeclampsia? _____ .

47. Rita George is hospitalized with severe preeclampsia. Identify five interventions commonly used in caring for a woman with preeclampsia and the rationale for each.

Intervention	Rationale
a.	
b.	
c.	
d.	
e.	

*48. Shortly after her admission to the hospital, Rita George begins crying and tells you she is worried that her preeclampsia will get worse and that she will have additional complications. She says, "I'm afraid I will never leave here alive." Based on this information, what nursing diagnosis would you formulate?

49. Rita is started on magnesium sulfate intravenously. Why?

50. Three symptoms of magnesium toxicity are _____ , _____ , and _____ .

51. a. The antagonist for magnesium sulfate is _____ .

    b. The correct dose is _____ by the _____ route.

52. A major hemorrhagic complication that may occur in women with severe preeclampsia is _____ .

*53. Identify at least four criteria that the nurse can use to evaluate the effectiveness of Rita's care.

    a.

    b.

    c.

    d.

54. Deborah Grand is admitted to the birthing center in active labor with her first pregnancy. Her blood pressure is now 140/86 (blood pressure at first prenatal visit was 110/66); she has 2+ pitting edema in her feet, ankles, and lower legs, and says that she has gained 4 pounds over the last 2 days.

   a. Describe the difference between 2+ and 4+ pitting edema.

   b. When you dipstick her urine for protein, you discover it is 3+. Why is this associated with pregnancy-induced hypertension (PIH)? What does this result mean?

   c. You check her deep tendon reflexes (DTR). The patella is usually used. What does 3+ DTR mean?

  *d. As you check DTR, you also assess clonus. How will you do this? What does 2 beats of clonus mean?

*55. A continuous IV of magnesium sulfate is ordered. Mrs Grand has respirations of 10, urine output of 25 mL/hr, and 1+ DTR with no clonus, and her blood pressure is 120/80. Do these findings indicate the expected outcome of the medical treatment? What treatment needs to be initiated now?

   a. You note that supplies have been gathered to protect Mrs Grand in case she has a convulsion. What supplies are important to have ready?

56. Describe the side effects the newborn might exhibit if the mother has been receiving IV magnesium sulfate in labor.

Rh Incompatibility

*57. The following situation has been developed to challenge your critical thinking. Read the situation and then answer the question "yes" or "no."

Your client, Carolyn Lorenzo, G2 P2, is Rh−; her partner is Rh+. Her first child was Rh−. She has just given birth to an Rh+ infant. Her indirect Coombs test is positive. Her infant's direct Coombs test is also positive.

Is Carolyn a candidate for RhIgG (RhoGAM)?
_____
                    ⇓   ⇓

Yes (Why? _____)   No (Why not? _____)

58. Explain RhoGAM, including what it is, when it is given, and how it works.

_____

*These questions are addressed at the end of Part I.

59. Briefly discuss the major risks for a woman and her fetus if the woman suffers trauma from an automobile accident during pregnancy.

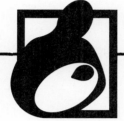

It's Your Turn

Think about a woman you have cared for or someone you have known whose pregnancy was considered high risk. What impact did it have on the woman and her family? How well did they cope? What actions by health care providers were helpful or not helpful?

_____

_____

_____

_____

_____

_____

_____

_____

_____

_____

_____

60. The TORCH infections pose a serious threat to pregnancy. For each of the following infections, identify the causative organism, maternal-fetal implications, treatment, and teaching:

Infection	Maternal-Fetal Implications	Treatment	Teaching

Toxoplasmosis

Cause:

Rubella

Cause:

Cytomegalovirus

Cause:

Herpesvirus type 2

Cause:

61. The following infections are also discussed in Chapter 3. Briefly summarize the implications of each for a pregnant woman or her fetus/neonate:

Moniliasis

Trichomoniasis

Chlamydia trachomatis

Syphilis

Gonorrhea

Condyloma accuminata

Lower urinary tract infection

Upper urinary tract infection

Selected Answers

This section addresses the asterisked questions found in this chapter.

6. Whenever possible, vaginal birth is preferred, using low forceps and a local or regional anesthetic to decrease the stress of the second stage of labor. This procedure also avoids the hazards associated with abdominal surgery for cesarean birth.

10. Belle Arthur did maintain effective control. Glycosylated hemoglobin is an accurate indicator of a person's long-term control. In the presence of elevated blood glucose levels, hemoglobin A_0 converts to hemoglobin A_{1c} or glycosylated hemoglobin. Since the process is essentially irreversible, elevations indicate that the person has been hyperglycemic. The normal range is approximately 6% to 8%. Thus, Ms Arthur's glycohemoglobin level of 7.0% is within normal limits.

11. An appropriate nursing diagnosis might be "Noncompliance with appointment schedule related to lack of adequate transportation."

12. Your intervention was very effective. You began by asking Ms Arthur for her opinion about ways of helping her keep her appointment. As is often the case, the client herself had obviously thought about the problem and tried to correct it but was unable to do so without assistance. By working in a collaborative way with Ms Arthur and the physician, you were able to arrange an effective solution. Good job!

14. Oral hypoglycemic agents are used in treating certain types of diabetes. However, because they have been linked to fetal abnormalities, they are contraindicated during pregnancy.

37. HCG levels are measured weekly, then bimonthly, and then monthly to monitor status. Elevated hCG titers may indicate the possible development of choriocarcinoma. Birth control, usually using the pill, is necessary, because it would be difficult to tell whether elevated hCG levels were related to pregnancy or to a developing malignancy.

38. a. Sarah Smythe is 36 years old and is a gravida 4. She has two children at home ; one of them was born at 35 weeks' gestation. Sarah had one spontaneous abortion. She smokes 10 cigarettes a day and has an occasional glass of wine. Sarah has a history of pyelonephritis. She has been working for the past 2 years in a factory. Her job requires that she stand in one place along a conveyor belt and inspect parts as they pass by. Sarah had a brief episode of vaginal bleeding at 14 weeks' gestation, which lasted 2 days. Since then, the pregnancy has gone well; however, she has noted more contractions lately.

Using Creasy, Gummer, and Liggins' system for determining risk of spontaneous preterm birth, factors in Sarah Smythe's history would receive the following points:

1 point each	Two children at home
	Works outside the home
	One spontaneous abortion
3 points each	Heavy work
4 points each	History of pyelonephritis
	Bleeding at 14 weeks
	Uterine irritability
10 points each	One previous preterm birth

b. To answer Mrs Smythe, you will need to include the following: She will need to watch for signs of preterm labor, which include uterine contractions every 10 minutes or less, mild menstrual-like cramps felt low in the abdomen, feelings of pelvic pressure, low backache that is constant or comes and goes, a change in vaginal discharge, abdominal cramping with or without diarrhea.

Teach her to lie down on her side or tilted to one side with a pillow. She may then place her fingertips on the fundus of the uterus. She checks for contractions (hardening or tightening) for about one hour. If contractions are felt every 10 minutes for one hour, she needs to call her health care provider.

c. A contraction will feel like a hardening or tightening of the uterus. She may also note a backache that comes and goes on a regular pattern of every 10 minutes. This may be associated with contractions.

39. Although the signs and symptoms of preterm labor are not clearly definitive, there are many subtle clues. You will probably need to place an "X" beside nausea, diarrhea, backache, and unusual tiredness.

40. c. 0.1 mg/min = 20 mL/hr

$$\frac{0.1 \text{ mg/min}}{20 \text{ mL/hr}} = \frac{0.35 \text{ mg/min}}{x \text{ mL/hr}}$$

$$0.1x = 7.00$$
$$x = 70 \text{ mL/hr}$$

41. c. She needs to know to take the medication on time, to observe for signs of preterm labor, and to assess her pulse with each dose. She will need to report a pulse above 120, palpitations, tremors, agitation, nervousness, chest pain, and/or any difficulty breathing.

43. a. Mrs Quick has a number of factors present that contraindicate beginning therapy to stop her labor. She is 5 cm dilated, and her contractions indicate active labor. Her membranes have been ruptured for just short of 24 hours, and although you do not know the cause of her low-grade fever, you should suspect amnionitis at this point.

These factors would lead you to answer "no." The most pressing nursing goal is probably to prepare for childbrith. With three previous births, a small baby this time (34 weeks' gestation), and 5 cm dilatation with active labor, the birth may be just a few minutes away.

b. (1) Use Nitrazine to test for ruptured membranes. It is important to establish whether membranes are ruptured; this needs to be done before any lubricant is used with a vaginal exam.

(2) Do a sterile vaginal exam to help gather data to determine if cervical effacement and dilatation have begun, and identify contraindications to treatment for preterm labor. The results of the exam may indicate you need to prepare for immediate birth.

(3) Apply the fetal monitor to obtain ongoing essential data.

(4) Assess maternal vital signs.

Items that are not essential at this time are completing all sections of the data form, obtaining her weight, and listening to breath sounds.

c. Mrs Golden

(1) Apply the EFM to provide data about the contraction pattern and fetal status. It is important to know fetal status prior to initiating ritodrine therapy and to provide ongoing information.

(2) Obtain maternal vital signs. This not only provides information regarding current status and provides a baseline, but also assists in identifying any contraindications to treatment (e.g., P above 120 may indicate cardiac problems, R above 24 may indicate respiratory problems, B/P above 140/90 may indicate hypertension).

(3) Prepare ritodrine therapy. This has been ordered STAT. However, the two preceding nursing actions should be prerequisites to this step.

Check out your ranking of these questions with your classmates, instructor, and nurses in the birth setting. If they agree, do they use the same rationale? If they disagree, ask them to share their thinking processes with you. There is not a "right" way to rank these. Conversations with others will bring insightful rewards.

44. *Actions:* We hope you would check Ms George's blood pressure and test her urine for protein.

Thoughts: Ms George's B/P is elevated significantly. An increase of 30/15 indicates mild preeclampsia. Ms George's B/P has increased 42/26, her urine contains protein, and she has had a major weight gain. Her symptoms indicate more than mild preeclampsia. We hope that at this point you would assess Rita for further signs of severe preeclampsia.

Assessments: At this point you could ask Ms George about additional symptoms such as headache, visual changes, or epigastric pain. You can quickly assess deep tendon reflexes and observe for evidence of edema.

Actions: You now have a clear picture of Ms George's status and should report your findings to the physician. Your preliminary assessments will help the physician realize the need to see Ms George quickly. Since you would expect the physician to admit Ms George to the hospital, you can quickly confirm his/her intentions and begin the necessary procedures for admission. You will thus avoid unnecessary delays for Ms George.

Thoughts: You know that the unexpected hospitalization must be stressful for Ms George. You also realize that she must have many questions and concerns.

Actions: Take the time to explain things to Ms George and answer her questions. She will probably be worried about the impact of the PIH on her unborn child and may also be worried about the problems caused for her family by her hospitalization. Having an opportunity to talk, plan, and consider her alternatives will be especially helpful. You can also offer to contact Ms George's family and explain the situation. If she is upset, it may be necessary to arrange with them to transport her to the hospital. Any support and assistance you can provide will be very helpful to her.

48. In light of Ms George's clearly expressed feelings, the most appropriate nursing diagnosis would be "Fear related to the risk of dying secondary to her diagnosed PIH."

53. Rita's care can be considered effective if the following criteria have been met:
a. Continued fetal well-being or birth of a healthy infant
b. Normal maternal blood pressure
c. Absence of proteinuria
d. Symptoms of preeclampsia/eclampsia controlled or absent
e. Mother able to resume activities of daily living
f. Mother able to care for infant (if born)

54. d. To assess clonus, the nurse quickly dorsoflexes the woman's foot. When there is hyperreflexia, the foot will jerk. Each movement (jerk) is counted, so 2 beats of clonus means there were two movements after the foot was dorsiflexed.

55. The factors listed indicate adverse effects of the IV magnesium sulfate therapy and not expected outcome of medical treatment. The dose of IV magnesium sulfate must be decreased to avoid a worsening of her condition.

57. If you answered "no" you were right on target. Carolyn Lorenzo is not a candidate for RhoGAM because her indirect Coombs test indicates that she has already been sensitized to Rh+ blood and has developed antibodies. Since her first baby was Rh− it is not known when Carolyn became sensitized. She may have had an undiagnosed pregnancy that ended in early miscarriage, she may have had a blood transfusion with Rh+ blood, or she may have had a small placental bleed during this pregnancy. Regardless of when it occurred, she needs a clear explanation of the risks she faces for hemolytic disease in subsequent pregnancies and her newborn needs to be evaluated carefully.

Part II Self-Assessment Guide

Do you know these abbreviations?

AIDS	CID
CMV	DIC
DM	DTR
FAS	GDM
HVH	IDDM
PIH	STD
TORCH	

Add your own abbreviations or new words you have learned:

Can you answer these questions?

The following multiple-choice questions will help you assess your knowledge of the content of this chapter. Select the best answer for each of the questions and then refer to the end of Part II to check your answers.

1. Which of the following statements about the nutritional needs of pregnant women with a cardiac condition is most accurate?
   a. They require major increases in iron and calories but decreased sodium.
   b. They require increased protein and iron but minimized sodium intake.
   c. They require optimal amounts of all essential vitamins but restricted caloric and iron intake.
   d. They require increased iron, protein, sodium, carbohydrates, and fats.

2. Vicky Brookens is at 34 weeks' gestation and is on intravenous ritodrine. She complains of nervousness. Her blood pressure has changed from 120/80 to 100/70. Her pulse rate is 154. Based on your knowledge of ritodrine, you will

    a. assess for bleeding because of the signs of impending shock.

    b. call the physician to report the decreased blood pressure and increased pulse.

    c. continue to follow your labor and birth protocol because all signs and symptoms are normal for ritodrine therapy.

    d. encourage Vicky to relax because her nervousness is affecting her vital signs.

3. Mary Lewis is pregnant for the second time. Her first child weighed 9 lb 11 oz. Her doctors perform a glucose tolerance test and discover elevated blood sugar levels. Because Mary shows no signs of diabetes when she is not pregnant, she is best classified as having

    a. type I diabetes mellitus.

    b. type II diabetes mellitus.

    c. gestational diabetes mellitus.

    d. secondary diabetes mellitus.

4. The major cause of spontaneous abortion is

    a. inadequate corpus luteum.

    b. placental inadequacies.

    c. reproductive tract defects.

    d. defects of the ovum or sperm.

5. Tamara Clarkson, at 11 weeks' gestation, calls her doctor and reports that she is having some mild vaginal bleeding and occasional mild cramps but no other problems. She is best characterized as having

    a. a threatened abortion.

    b. a missed abortion.

    c. an imminent abortion.

    d. an incomplete abortion.

6. Which of the following signs would *not* be indicative of a ruptured tubal pregnancy?

    a. Marked lower abdominal pain

    b. Vaginal bleeding

    c. Urinary frequency

    d. Increased pulse and decreased blood pressure

7. Women with a diagnosis of severe preeclampsia have an increased risk of

    a. complete abortion.

    b. placenta previa.

    c. abruptio placentae.

    d. none of the above.

8. You are administering intravenous magnesium sulfate to a woman with severe preeclampsia. You assess her and find respirations 12, DTRs (deep tendon reflexes) absent, urine output for the past 4 hours of 90 mL. What would you do?

    a. Administer calcium gluconate immediately.

    b. Administer only half the dose of magnesium sulfate.

    c. Continue the magnesium sulfate as ordered.

    d. Stop the magnesium sulfate and notify the doctor.

9. Thrush in the newborn is directly related to contact in the birth canal with which of the following organisms?
   a. *Candida albicans*
   b. *Neisseria gonorrhoeae*
   c. *Treponema pallidum*
   d. *Staphylococcus aureus*

10. In order to protect her unborn child from toxoplasmosis, a pregnant woman should
    a. avoid contact with people known to have German measles.
    b. avoid eating inadequately cooked meat.
    c. avoid sexual relations with known carriers of the causative organism.
    d. be vaccinated against it early in her pregnancy.

11. Which of the following findings would best support a diagnosis of gestational trophoblastic disease?
    a. Elevated hCG levels, enlarged abdomen, quickening
    b. Vaginal bleeding, absence of fetal heart tones, decreased hCG levels
    c. Visible fetal skeleton with sonography, absence of quickening, enlarged abdomen
    d. Brownish vaginal discharge, hyperemesis gravidarum, absence of fetal heart tones

Answers

1. b	2. c	3. c	4. d	5. a	6. c
7. c	8. d	9. a	10. b	11. d	

8

Fetal Assessment

Introduction

Nurses have an important role in fetal assessment. The nurse frequently provides the one-on-one teaching regarding the purpose, procedure, and possible alternatives of each fetal test. The nurse is able to interpret test results and assist the couple in understanding the test.

This chapter addresses the diagnostic testing that may be done during the prenatal period. This chapter corresponds to Chapter 20 in *Maternal-Newborn Nursing: A Family-Centered Approach,* 4th ed.

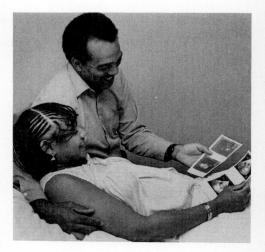

Part I Concepts, Critical Thinking, and Clinical Applications

*1. Identify at least three conditions in which it will be very important to assess the fetus during the prenatal period. Why is it important to assess these conditions?

2. Sylvia Parker is scheduled for chorionic villus sampling (CVS).

   a. At what point in the gestation will this most likely be done?

   b. Summarize the benefits and risks for the mother and fetus.

   c. During the procedure, what type of tissue is obtained and what tests may be done?

   d. Explain the information that may be discovered as a result of the CVS.

   e. Identify three essential elements of a teaching plan you will develop for Sylvia.

---

*These questions are addressed at the end of Part I.

Ultrasound

*3. List two advantages for the mother and fetus of using ultrasound for assessment.

   a.

   b.

4. Identify at least six uses of ultrasound during early and late pregnancy.

Early Pregnancy (to 24 weeks)	Late Pregnancy (over 36 weeks)

   a.

   b.

   c.

   d.

   e.

   f.

5. Mrs Blythe Coleman is having an ultrasound examination. She asks, "Is it safe for my baby?" What will you say?

6. Hazel Applegate, Gr 3 P 1, is in her 23rd week of pregnancy. Her last normal menstrual period began 5 1/2 months ago, but she had some bleeding 4 1/2 months ago. Your physical assessment provides the following data: The fundus is palpable at two fingerbreadths below the umbilicus; the fetal heart rate (FHR) is 140. Hazel states that she has not felt quickening. Based on this information, why do you think Hazel will have an ultrasound done?

7. Hazel asks you what is involved in having an ultrasound. How will you respond?

*These questions are addressed at the end of Part I.

Maternal Assessment of Fetal Activity

8. Carla Lewis is pregnant for the first time. She asks you how to monitor her baby's movements.

   a. Write out your teaching plan.

   b. In the space below, devise a score sheet that she could use.

   c. She asks if there is anything she can do that might affect the number of movements. How will you answer?

Nonstress Testing

9. What is the function of a nonstress test (NST)?

10. Explain the procedure for performing an NST.

11. Fetal heart rate patterns in NSTs have four classifications. Describe what a fetal monitoring strip would show in each case. What further testing may be indicated?

    a. Reactive

    b. Nonreactive

    c. Unsatisfactory

12. What is the best test result? Why?

*13. Label each section of Figure 8–1A and B as reactive, nonreactive, or unsatisfactory.

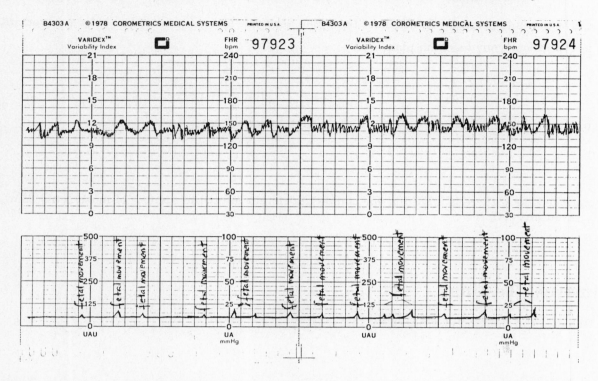

Figure 8–1A _____

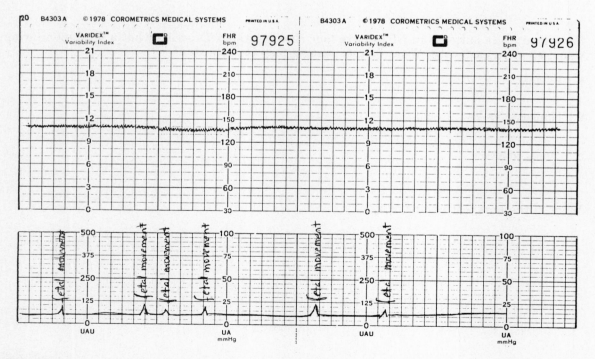

Figure 8–1B _____

---

*These questions are addressed at the end of Part I.

14. This tracing (Figure 8–1C) depicts a suspicious NST. In colored pen or pencil, draw over the pattern and change it to a reactive pattern.

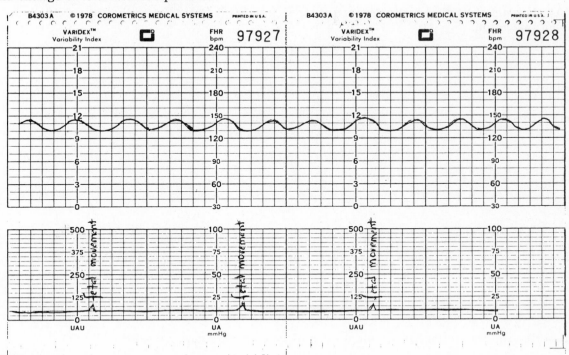

Figure 8–1C

15. The NST can be modified by adding a fetal acoustic stimulation test (FAST). Describe how the FAST changes the basic NST.

Biophysical Profile

16. A biophysical profile is completed to assess the fetus.

    a. Discuss the specific areas assessed in this test.

    b. How is it scored? What represents a "desirable" or "good" score?

    c. Describe the conditions in which it is most likely for a fetal biophysical profile to be done.

    d. What does a small pocket of fluid mean?

    e. Mr Robinson calls the birth center and says "My wife is to have a fetal biophysical profile tomorrow. What is it?" Write out how you will describe the assessment test for him.

Contraction Stress Testing

*17. List six indications for doing a contraction stress test (CST). Describe the physiologic rationale behind each indication.

a.

b.

c.

d.

e.

f.

*18. List three contraindications for the CST. Describe the physiologic rationale behind each.

19. Describe the procedure for the nipple stimulation contraction stress-test (NSCST).

20. Explain the major differences between NSCST and CST with intravenous oxytocin (sometimes called oxytocin challenge test).

21. Describe the procedure for NSCST.

22. Write out the exact words you would use to explain each CST result. As you think about your answer, visualize the woman or couple you would be talking to and include a description. Make something about this couple stand out so the words will stay with you.

23. Write out the exact words you would use to explain a reactive and a nonreactive NST. Again personalize the situation with real people.

*These questions are addressed at the end of Part I.

24. *a. Label the two CST tracings in Figure 8–2A and B as positive or negative.

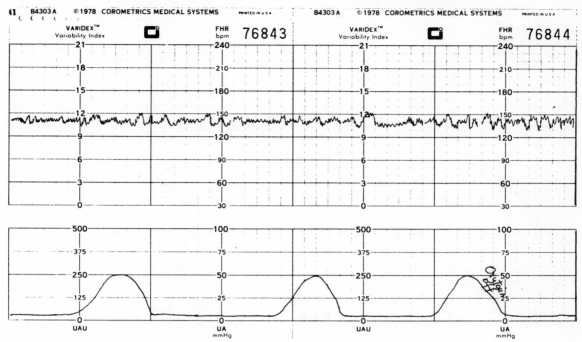

Figure 8–2A _____

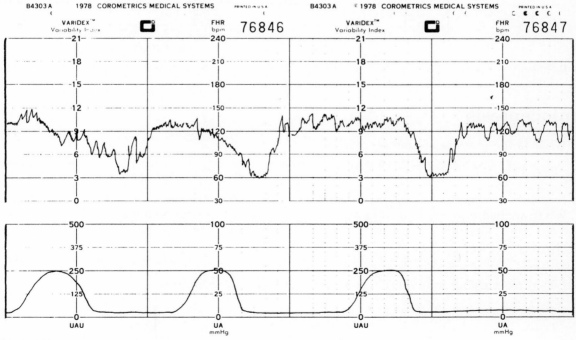

Figure 8–2B _____

b. What factors led you to this conclusion?

---

*These questions are addressed at the end of Part I.

25. On the next tracing (Figure 8–3), draw your own test results. Use different colored ink so the tracings will stand out.

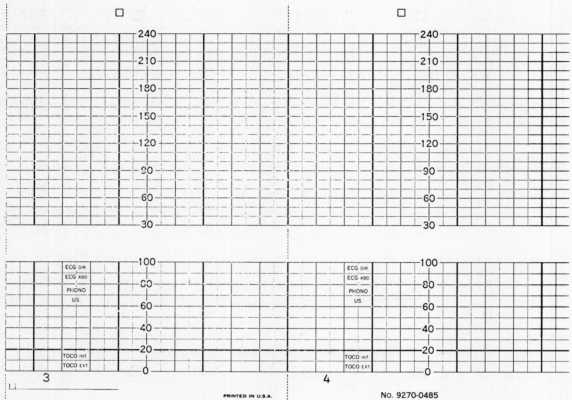

Figure 8–3

Amniocentesis

26. What is the purpose of amniocentesis?

27. What method may be used to locate the placenta prior to amniocentesis?

*28. List three nursing interventions necessary during amniocentesis.

29. List three complications associated with amniocentesis.

    a.

    b.

    c.

---

*These questions are addressed at the end of Part I.

30. Complete the chart on various tests that may be performed on amniotic fluid in the later portion of pregnancy.

Test	Purpose of Test	Normal Results	What Results Mean
(L/S) Lecithin/ Sphingomyelin Ratio			
Prostaglandin			
Creatinine			

*31. **Action Sequence**
Holly Swit, a 37-year-old primipara, had an amniocentesis today. Holly calls the antepartal testing room 5 hours after her amniocentesis and says she is having contractions. Holly is 38 weeks' gestation.

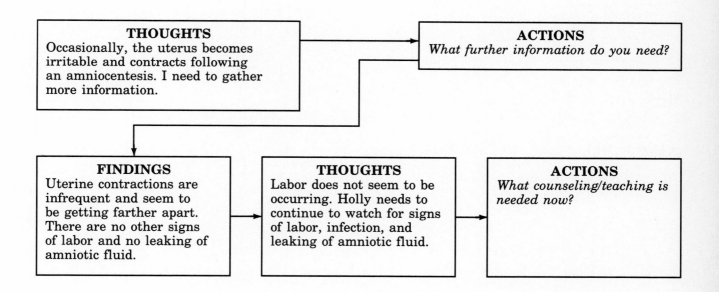

THOUGHTS
Occasionally, the uterus becomes irritable and contracts following an amniocentesis. I need to gather more information.

ACTIONS
What further information do you need?

FINDINGS
Uterine contractions are infrequent and seem to be getting farther apart. There are no other signs of labor and no leaking of amniotic fluid.

THOUGHTS
Labor does not seem to be occurring. Holly needs to continue to watch for signs of labor, infection, and leaking of amniotic fluid.

ACTIONS
What counseling/teaching is needed now?

*These questions are addressed at the end of Part I.

*32. The following situation has been developed to challenge your critical thinking. Read the situation and then answer the question "yes" or "no."

Your client, Amy Blankin, is a 15-year-old gravida 1 who is in her 35th week of pregnancy. An amniocentesis is done to assess fetal lung maturity. Test results indicate an L/S ratio of 2:1 and prostaglandin (PG) is present.

Is fetal lung maturity indicated?

⇓   ⇓

YES   NO
(Explain your answer)   (Explain your answer)

---

*These questions are addressed at the end of Part I.

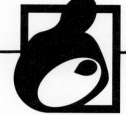

It's Your Turn

Talk with a pregnant woman who is having prenatal testing done. What are her needs, concerns, and fears? Did she understand the reason for the test and what the test results mean? Did she know what to expect? What advice does she have for nurses who work in the antepartal testing situation?

_____

_____

_____

_____

_____

_____

_____

_____

_____

_____

_____

_____

Selected Answers

This section addresses the asterisked questions found in this chapter.

1. An evaluation of fetal status may be needed in the presence of any of the following:
   a. Failure of the uterus to enlarge at the expected rate or accelerated enlargement
   b. Failure to auscultate fetal heart beat
   c. Medical complications during pregnancy, such as diabetes and preeclampsia-eclampsia
   d. Problems with previous pregnancies, such as fetal death, premature infant, and intrauterine growth retardation (IUGR)

   This list is not all-inclusive but does identify some major factors. If you had difficulty with this question, you should review prenatal complications in your textbook.

3. Some advantages of ultrasound testing are that
   a. it is noninvasive.
   b. it is a painless procedure with the exception of discomfort from a full bladder and from having to lie on one's back for a while.
   c. there is no radiation involved, as with x rays.
   d. no specific ill effects are now known.
   e. it allows for differentiation of soft tissue.
   f. immediate information can be gained.

13. Figure 8–1A is reactive; B is nonreactive.

17. Indications for a CST include the following:
   a. IUGR
   b. Diabetes mellitus
   c. Heart disease
   d. Preeclampsia-eclampsia
   e. Sickle cell disease
   f. Suspected postmaturity
   g. History of previous stillborn
   h. Rh sensitization
   i. Abnormal estriol excretion
   j. Hyperthyroidism
   k. Renal disease

18. Contraindications for a CST include the following:
   a. Third-trimester bleeding
   b. Previous cesarean birth
   c. Instances in which the possible risk of premature labor outweighs the advantages of the CST

24. a. Figure 8–2A is a negative CST; B is a positive CST.

28. Nursing interventions during an amniocentesis should include the following:
   a. Prepare the equipment.
   b. Cleanse the abdomen.
   c. Assess the maternal vital signs and the FHR prior to amniocentesis and after the procedure is completed.
   d. Document amniocentesis in the client's chart.
   e. Provide information and support to the client.

31. *Action:* You need to know more about the contraction characteristics (such as frequency, duration, and intensity of contractions) and if there are any additional signs of labor.

   Action: You will need to reiterate the discharge instructions, which should include signs of labor, how to assess uterine contractions, and signs of infections.

32. The correct answer is YES. Did you select that one? The L/S ratio is mature and the presence of PG is also associated with fetal lung maturity.

Part II Self-Assessment Guide

Do you know these abbreviations?

AC	BPP	BSST	CRL	CST	AFV
FAST	FBM	FBPP	FL	HC	IUGR
NSCST	NST	US	VST		

Add your own abbreviations or new words that you have learned:

Can you answer these questions?

The following multiple-choice questions will help you assess your knowledge of the content of this chapter. Select the best answer for each of the questions and then refer to the end of Part II to check your answers.

1. An ultrasound reading is done prior to amniocentesis to
   a. avoid any large pockets of amniotic fluid.
   b. decide if the fetus is mature enough.
   c. determine fetal lung maturity.
   d. locate the placenta.

2. Immediately after amniocentesis is completed, the expectant mother complains of dizziness and shortness of breath. Which of the following would best explain the cause?
   a. Pressure of the physician's hands while he or she was withdrawing fluid
   b. Pressure of the uterus on the vena cava while the woman has been lying on her back
   c. The size of the needle that was used
   d. The normal result of having amniotic fluid withdrawn from the uterus

3. A woman calls back 2 hours after having amniocentesis done. She reports that she is having contractions every 5 minutes and is leaking clear fluid. Your best response is that
   a. this is a normal result of amniocentesis.
   b. she should notify her physician and proceed to the birth unit.
   c. she should rest and call back in 8 hours if the contractions have not subsided.
   d. she should time her contractions for 4 hours and then call the physician.

4. A woman has had several diagnostic tests done in the past 2 days. The results are BPD 9.5 cm; creatinine 2 mg/dL; L/S 2.5:1. If birth occurs today, you know that
   a. she will have a term infant.
   b. she may have twins.
   c. she will have a stillborn fetus.
   d. you should alert a pediatrician and the intensive care nursery to expect a preterm infant.

5. A CST would most likely be done for a woman who has
   a. a fetal L/S ratio of 1.5:1.
   b. a nonreactive NST.
   c. had amniocentesis for genetic assessment.
   d. had twins.

6. The results of a CST show three contractions in 10 minutes without late decelerations. The CST is
   a. negative.
   b. positive.
   c. suspicious.
   d. unsatisfactory and must be reported.

7. An example of a sex chromosome abnormality is
   a. Down syndrome.
   b. Tay-Sachs disease
   c. Trisomy 13.
   d. Turner syndrome.

Answers

1. d   2. b   3. b   4. a   5. b   6. a   7. d

Birth: Stages and Processes

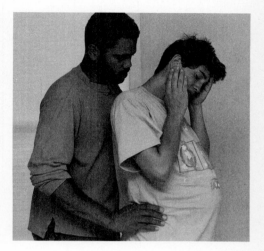

Introduction

Successful labor and birth result from the effective interplay of anatomic, physiologic, and psychologic factors. This chapter considers the role of each of these factors in the process of birth. It begins with pertinent terminology and focuses on significant aspects of physiologic and psychologic changes. It then focuses on the mechanisms of labor and the stages into which labor is divided.

This chapter corresponds to Chapter 21 in *Maternal-Newborn Nursing: A Family-Centered Approach,* 4th ed.

Part I Concepts, Critical Thinking, and Clinical Applications

Maternal Pelvis

1. List the four Caldwell-Moloy types of pelves and include a drawing of the basic shape of each type.

   a.

   b.

   c.

   d.

2. Complete the following chart:

Pelvic Type	Incidence	Major Characteristics of:			Implications for Labor and Birth
		Inlet	Midpelvis	Outlet	
Gynecoid					
Android					
Anthropoid					
Platypelloid					

The Fetus

3. Label the parts of the fetal skull indicated in Figure 9–1.

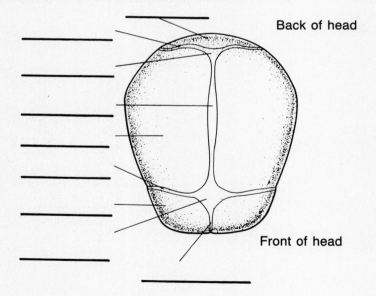

Back of head

Front of head

Figure 9–1 Superior view of the fetal skull.

4. Define *suture.*

5. Describe the location of the following:
    a. Mitotic (frontal) suture

    b. Sagittal suture

    c. Coronal suture

    d. Lambdoidal suture

6. Define *fontanelle*. Why are fontanelles important in the fetal skull?

7. Describe the location and characteristic size of the following:
    a. Anterior fontanelle

    b. Posterior fontanelle

8. Label the landmarks of the fetal skull indicated on Figure 9–2.

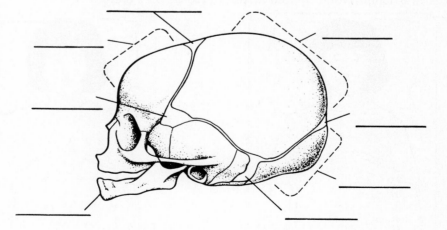

Figure 9–2 Lateral view of the fetal skull.

9. Figure 9–3 depicts the anteroposterior and transverse diameters of the fetal head. Label each of the diameters and state the "norms" for an average size full-term newborn.

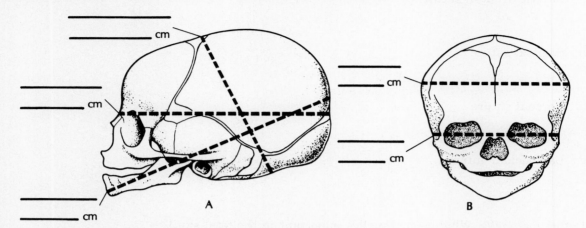

Figure 9–3   **A.** Anteroposterior diameters of the fetal skull.   **B.** Transverse diameters of the fetal skull.

10. Define *fetal attitude*.

11. Define *fetal position*. How does it differ from fetal attitude?

12. Define *fetal lie*.

13. Draw a fetus in a longitudinal lie and a transverse lie on Figure 9–4.

A.
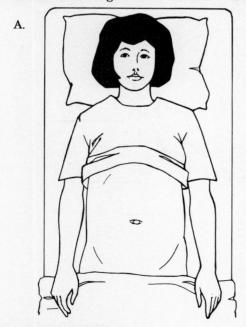

B.
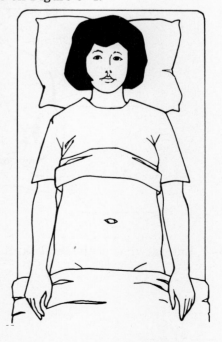

Figure 9–4 Fetal position.
A. Longitudinal lie. **B.** Transverse lie.

14. Define *fetal presentation.*

15. List the four types of cephalic presentation.

    a.

    b.

    c.

    d.

16. List and describe the three types of breech presentation. Explain how they are different.

    a.

    b.

    c.

*17. Label the fetal presentations and positions shown in Figure 9–5.

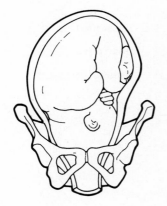 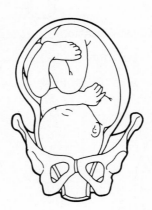 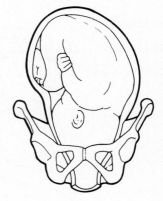

A. presentation _____

    position _____

    presenting part _____

B. presentation _____

    position _____

    presenting part _____

C. presentation _____

    position _____

    presenting part _____

Continued

*These questions are addressed at the end of Part I.

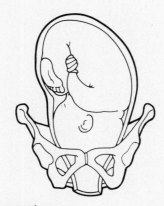
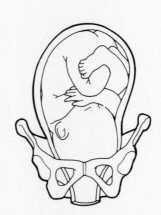
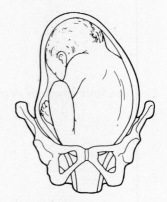

D. presentation _____
   position _____
   presenting part _____

E. presentation _____
   position _____
   presenting part _____

F. presentation _____
   position _____
   presenting part _____

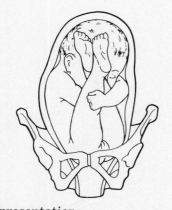
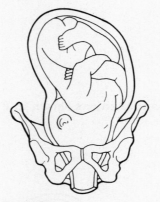
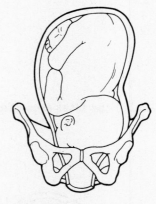

G. presentation _____
   position _____
   presenting part _____

H. presentation _____
   position _____
   presenting part _____

I. presentation _____
   position _____
   presenting part _____

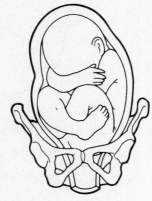
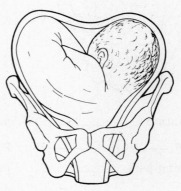

J. presentation_____
   position _____
   presenting part _____

K. presentation _____
   position _____
   presenting part _____

Continued

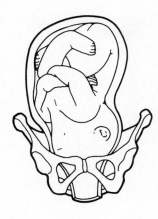

L. presentation _____

     position _____

     presenting part _____

M. presentation _____

     position _____

     presenting part _____

Figure 9–5

*18. List three methods that could be used to determine presentation and position.

     a.

     b.

     c.

19. Define *engagement*.

20. When does engagement generally occur

     a. for a primigravida?

     b. for a multigravida?

     c. How is engagement determined?

_____

*These questions are addressed at the end of Part I.

*21. What information does engagement provide about adequacy of the midpelvis or outlet?

*22. Describe two methods used to determine engagement.

   a.

   b.

23. What does the term "floating" or "ballotable" mean?

*24. Devise two questions you could ask the expectant mother that would elicit information about symptoms indicative of engagement. Include your rationale.

   a.

   b.

25. Define *station*.

26. How is station assessed?

27. Explain what a −1 station is.

Uterine Contractions

28. Draw a line between the term in column one and the correct definition in column two.

   Column One   Column Two

   a. Acme   _____ The building up of the contraction

   b. Decrement   _____ The letting up of the contraction

   c. Duration   _____ The peak of the contraction

   d. Frequency   _____ From the beginning of one to the beginning of the next contraction

   e. Increment   _____ The time from the beginning to the end of one contraction

   f. Intensity   _____ The strength of the contraction

---

*These questions are addressed at the end of Part I.

29. Label each of the areas indicated in Figure 9–6.

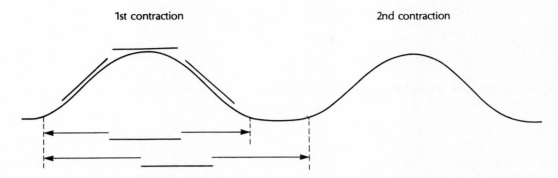

Figure 9–6 Characteristics of uterine contractions.

Psychologic State

30. Identify the factors that may affect a woman's psychologic response to labor.

31. Describe how a woman's cultural background might affect her psychologic status in labor.

Physiology of Labor

32. Describe each of the following premonitory signs of labor:

    a. Lightening

    b. Braxton Hicks contractions

    c. Cervical changes

    d. Bloody show

    e. Rupture of membranes

    f. Increase in energy

33. The factors that initiate labor are not known, but there are some current theories. Discuss each of the following:

    a. Oxytocin stimulation theory

    b. Progesterone withdrawal theory

c. Estrogen stimulation theory

d. Fetal cortisol theory

e. Fetal membrane phospholipid–arachidonic acid–prostaglandin theory

34. The positional changes of the fetus during labor are termed *mechanisms of labor* or *cardinal movements*. Describe each of the following components of this process for a vertex presentation:

a. Descent and engagement

b. Flexion

c. Internal rotation

d. Extension

e. Restitution and external rotation

f. Expulsion

35. Labor and birth are divided into four stages, each with a definite beginning and ending. Complete the following chart:

Stage	Begins	Ends
First		
Second		
Third		
Fourth		

36. The first stage of labor is divided into which three phases?

   a.

   b.

   c.

37. Complete the following chart:

Characteristics of Labor	First Stage: Latent Phase	First Stage: Active Phase	First Stage: Transition Phase	Second Stage	Third Stage
Average duration for primigravida					
Average duration for multigravida					
Frequency of contractions					

Continued

Characteristics of Labor	First Stage: Latent Phase	First Stage: Active Phase	First Stage: Transition Phase	Second Stage	Third Stage
Duration of contractions					
Intensity of contractions					
Cervical dilatation					

38. Complete the following chart of maternal and fetal reponses to labor:

System	Expected Changes	Physiologic Rationale
Maternal cardiovascular		
Maternal respiratory		

Continued

System	Expected Changes	Physiologic Rationale
Maternal renal		
Maternal gastrointestinal		
Maternal hemopoietic		
Fetal cardiovascular		

Psychosocial/Cultural Adaptations to Labor

39. Discuss some possible psychologic responses to the birthing process.

40. Describe the "normal" psychologic response to each phase of the first stage of labor.

    a. Latent phase

    b. Active phase

    c. Transition phase

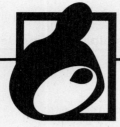

It's Your Turn

Frequently the experience of labor is much different from the "norms" that textbooks address because each individual is different. What was your labor or the labor of a client like? Did it match the characteristics that you are learning about now? How was it different?

_____

_____

_____

_____

_____

_____

_____

_____

_____

_____

_____

_____

_____

_____

_____

_____

_____

_____

_____

Selected Answers

This section addresses the asterisked questions found in this chapter.

17. The answers to this question have been provided because some students have difficulty in determining presentation and position.

    a. Cephalic presentation; ROA; presenting part-occiput

    b. Cephalic presentation; LOP; presenting part-occiput

    c. Cephalic presentation; LOA; presenting part-occiput

    d. Cephalic presentation; LOT; presenting part-occiput

    e. Cephalic presentation; ROP; presenting part-occiput

    f. Breech presentation; LSA; presenting part-sacrum

    g. Breech presentation; RSA; presenting part-sacrum

    h. Cephalic (face) presentation; LMA; presenting part-mentum

    i. Cephalic (face) presentation; RMP; presenting part-mentum

    j. Breech presentation; LSP; presenting part-sacrum

    k. Transverse lie; LAPA; presenting part-shoulder

    l. Cephalic (face) presentation; RMA; presenting part-mentum

    m. Breech presentation; single footling; presenting part-single footling

    If you had difficulty with this question, refer back to the definitions of presentation and position. It may also help to use a model of a pelvis with a fetus. This is an important concept to grasp, so keep at it.

18. Methods used to determine fetal presentation and position include

    a. Leopold's maneuvers.

    b. visual inspection of the maternal abdomen.

    c. location of the fetal heart tones.

    d. vaginal examination.

    e. assessment of the mother's greatest area of discomfort (for example, a fetus in the posterior position tends to cause more low back pain).

    f. visualization by ultrasound.

21. None. Engagement provides information about the inlet but not about the midpelvis or outlet. Fetal descent would provide information about the midpelvis and outlet.

22. Leopold's maneuvers and vaginal examinations can be used to determine engagement. X-ray pelvimetry would also provide this information but would not be used solely to determine engagement of the fetal head.

24. The questions should be directed toward changes the mother might feel once engagement has occurred.

   a. "Have you recently noticed a change in the way your clothes fit?" Rationale: As the fetal head drops into the inlet, there may be a change in the shape of the abdomen. It may seem that the baby has dropped down and away from the mother's body. This causes a change in the way her clothes fit.

   b. "Have you recently noticed that you have to urinate more frequently?" Rationale: As the fetus descends into the pelvis, there may be more pressure on the bladder.

   c. "Have you noticed more discomfort in your pelvic area and your thighs?" Rationale: As the fetus decends into the pelvis, there may be more discomfort. There may also be increased pressure from vasocongestion of the areas below the pelvis (that is, the perineum and the lower extremities).

   d. "Have you noticed easier breathing?" Rationale: As the fetus descends into the pelvis, there may be less pressure on the diaphragm.

   Any of these changes may suggest that engagement has occurred, but they are not diagnostic.

Part II Self-Assessment Guide

Do you know these abbreviations?

LADA	LOT	ROA
LADP	LSA	ROM
LMA	LSP	ROP
LMP	LST	ROT
LMT	RMA	RSA
LOA	RMP	RSP
LOP	RMT	RST

Do you know the following words?

acme	decrement
bloody show	fontanelles
Braxton Hicks	increment
cardinal movements	lightening
crowning	premonitory

Add your own abbreviations or new words that you have learned:

Can you answer these questions?

The following multiple-choice questions will help you assess your knowledge of the content of this chapter. Select the best answer for each of the questions and then refer to the end of Part II to check your answers.

1. A typical gynecoid pelvis would have which of the following characteristics?
    a. Rounded inlet, nonprominent ischial spines, and wide, round pubic arch
    b. Heart-shaped inlet, prominent ischial spines, and narrow, deep pubic arch
    c. Oval outlet, prominent or nonprominent ischial spines, and normal or moderately narrow pubic arch
    d. Transverse oval inlet, prominent or nonprominent ischial spines, and wide pubic arch

2. At term you would expect the suboccipitobregmatic diameter of the fetal head to be approximately
    a. 8 cm.
    b. 9.5 cm.
    c. 11.75 cm.
    d. 13.5 cm.

3. Engagement of the presenting part occurs when the largest diameter of the presenting part
    a. begins to enter the pelvic inlet but can be dislodged with gentle pressure.
    b. is level with the ischial spines.
    c. passes through the pelvic inlet.
    d. passes through the pelvic outlet.

4. A cephalic presentation includes all of the following *except*
    a. brow.
    b. face.
    c. shoulder.
    d. vertex.

5. Which of the following are considered premonitory signs of labor?
    a. Bloody show, desire to bear down
    b. Desire to bear down, increased vaginal secretions
    c. Lightening, increased vaginal secretions
    d. Rupture of membranes, elevated temperature

6. It is often difficult to distinguish true labor from false labor. In false labor,
    a. contractions are of variable frequency and are relieved by walking.
    b. contractions are felt primarily in the lower back.
    c. contractions increase in frequency, duration, and intensity with progressive cervical dilatation.
    d. contractions seem to start in the back and radiate around the abdomen in a girdlelike fashion.

7. To determine frequency, uterine contractions are timed from the
    a. beginning of one contraction to the beginning of the next.
    b. end of one contraction to the beginning of the next.
    c. end of one contraction to the end of the next contraction.
    d. beginning of one contraction to the end of that contraction.

8. There are various theories regarding the cause of labor onset. One possible cause involves
   a. an increase in the amount of circulating progesterone.
   b. a decrease in the amount of circulating estrogen.
   c. production of endogenous oxytocin by the mother's pituitary gland.
   d. inactivation of phospholipase A_2.

9. The fetus adapts to the birth canal by undergoing some positional changes. Which of the following answers best describe the correct sequence?
   a. Descent and flexion, extension, internal rotation, external rotation
   b. Extension, descent and flexion, internal rotation, external rotation
   c. Internal rotation, descent and flexion, extension, external rotation
   d. Descent and flexion, internal rotation, extension, external rotation

10. A number of assessments may be made while performing a vaginal examination during labor. Which of the following is *least* likely to be determined at this time?
   a. Cervical dilatation
   b. Station
   c. Fetal descent
   d. Diagnosis of twins

Answers

1. a   2. b   3. c   4. c   5. c   6. a
7. a   8. c   9. d   10. d

Nursing Assessment and Care of the Intrapartal Family

10

Introduction

The intrapartal period marks the completion of pregnancy and the beginning of a new life. It is frequently referred to as a crisis; it is certainly a time of stress, as all aspects of the laboring woman—physiologic and psychologic—are affected.

Today, the birthing nurse must have a thorough understanding of the stages and processes of labor and the ability to correlate that knowledge with observable behavior and changes in the laboring woman and those supporting her. In essence, the nurse's understanding of labor and birth forms the basis for ongoing assessment, intervention, and evaluation of care during labor and birth.

This chapter emphasizes assessment, anticipated findings and their significance, and appropriate nursing interventions. Questions related to evaluation are also included to provide guidelines for determining the effectiveness of care. This chapter corresponds to Chapters 22, 23, and 24 in *Maternal-Newborn Nursing: A Family-Centered Approach,* 4th ed.

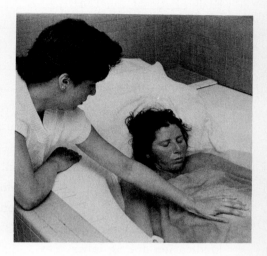

Part I Concepts, Critical Thinking, and Clinical Applications

1. List at least six intrapartal problems that would contribute to a woman being designated "high risk." Correlate each high-risk factor with the maternal and fetal newborn implications.

    a.

    b.

    c.

    d.

    e.

    f.

2. The following questionnaire is similar to many that are used when a woman is admitted to the labor and birth unit. Have a friend or family member act as a client and role-play a situation in which you, as the labor and birth nurse, complete the interview. (Note: This questionnaire focuses primarily on baseline information and does not include information that would require physical assessment.)

Admission date _____ Time _____ Admitting nurse _____

Patient name _____ Age _____

EDB _____ LMP _____ Length of gestation by dates _____

Attending MD/CNM_____ Pediatrician_____

Gravida _____ Para _____ Ab _____ Living children _____

Onset of labor: Spontaneous _____ Induced _____ Time _____ Bleeding _____

Membrane status: Intact _____ Ruptured _____ Time _____

Blood type _____ Rh _____ Serology _____ Date of serology of testing _____

Persons for maternal support during birth _____

Prenatal education classes: Yes _____ No _____ Type _____

Birthing requests: Feeding method: Breast _____ Bottle _____ Glucose water _____

Prep: Yes _____ No _____ Enema: Yes _____ No _____ Ambulation: Yes _____ No _____

Shower: Yes _____ No _____ Jacuzzi: Yes _____ No _____ Fetal monitor: Yes _____ No _____

Own choices of labor position: Yes _____ No _____ Birthing position: _____

Medication during labor: Yes _____ No _____ Regional block: Yes _____ No _____

Birth requests: _____

Other: _____

Prepregnancy weight _____ Present weight _____ Weight gain _____

Allergy: Medications _____ Foods _____ Substances _____

Time of last food intake _____ Type _____ Fluids _____

Medical problems prior to pregnancy _____

Problems with last pregnancy _____

Problems with this pregnancy _____

*3. Allison Scott is admitted to the birthing center accompanied by her husband, Craig. She is in early labor. During your initial interview, you discover that she is a primigravida and that her expected date of birth (EDB) is today. She has not attended prenatal classes. What four observations will you make while assessing her contractions?

a.

b.

c.

d.

4. Why do you use your fingertips instead of the palm of your hand to palpate contractions?

---

*These questions are addressed at the end of Part I.

5. What would you expect Allison's contractions to be like if she is in the latent phase?

6. The charge nurse records Allison's contractions as every 5 minutes, lasting 30 seconds, and of mild intensity.

   a. What is the frequency? _____

   b. What is the duration? _____

   c. What is the intensity? _____

*7. Craig hands you a piece of paper with a recording of contractions prior to admission. The paper shows:

CONTRACTION BEGINS	CONTRACTION ENDS
0500:00	0500:40
0505:00	0505:40
0508:00	0508:45
0511:00	0511:45

   What is the frequency of the contractions? _____

   What is the duration of the contractions? _____

8. What differences would you perceive when palpating mild, moderate, and strong (intense) contractions?

   a. Mild

   b. Moderate

   c. Strong

9. You will use a fetoscope to assess fetal heart rate (FHR).

   a. Describe the method you will use to locate the FHR.

   b. After locating the fetal heartbeat and just before counting the FHR, you check Allison's radial pulse. Explain the rationale for this.

   *c. How long should you listen to the FHR? At what times will it be important to assess FHR?

*10. As part of your assessment, you perform Leopold's maneuvers on Allison. How should she be positioned?

---

*These questions are addressed at the end of Part I.

*11. When you do Leopold's maneuvers, you feel a firm, rounded object in the uterine fundus; a smooth surface along the right side of the uterus (mother's right side); a surface that feels more nodular on the left side of the uterus; and a body part that is rounded and even more firm just above the symphysis. The fetal presentation is _____. The fetal position is _____ .

12. Identify one advantage of performing Leopold's maneuvers prior to locating the FHR.

*13. Explain why membrane status should be ascertained before a vaginal examination is done.

14. What effect do intact membranes have on labor progress?

15. Explain the implications of ruptured membranes for the mother and fetus.

*16. Why do you need to know the exact time that the membranes rupture?

17. Explain why the FHR is assessed immediately after the membranes have ruptured.

18. Explain nursing assessments and nursing care required when the woman has ruptured amniotic membranes. Write out the dialogue you would use in teaching the woman about ruptured membranes and about what to expect from the nurses.

19. Allison says she doesn't think she wants her membranes ruptured artificially, but she's not sure. She asks, "What do you think I should do?" Write out your answer. Remember, because you want to help her be an informed consumer, your answer needs to include assessment of Allison's knowledge and understanding, an overview of the purpose of amniotomy, advantages, disadvantages, and any known alternatives to the amniotomy.

*These questions are addressed at the end of Part I.

*20. To practice your role as client advocate, imagine you have just carefully explained an amniotomy to a woman, and she decides she doesn't want it done. The physician calls in and says "I'm on my way to the birthing unit to see Mrs X. I'm planning to do an amniotomy if all is going well." What will your response be?

*21. While examining Mrs X, the physician says, "Hand me an amnihook so I can rupture these membranes." Mrs X quickly looks to you, shaking her head from side to side. What will you say?

*22. Allison states that she is losing some clear fluid from her vagina when she coughs. You note that the Nitrazine test tape does not change color.

    a. Are the membranes intact or ruptured?

    b. What do you think the source of the clear fluid is?

23. You do a vaginal examination on Allison.

    *a. List the information that can be ascertained by performing a vaginal examination.

    b. How do you position Allison for the vaginal examination? What will you do to protect her privacy?

    c. Define *cervical dilatation*. How is dilatation recorded?

    d. Define *cervical effacement*. How is effacement recorded?

---

*These questions are addressed at the end of Part I.

24. During the vaginal examination, you find that you can place two fingers side by side in Allison's cervix. You can feel a firm surface against the cervix and a softer triangular shape in the upper right position (between 12 and 3 on a clock). You also note a small amount of bloody show.

    *a. What is the cervical dilatation?

    *b. What is the presentation?

    *c. What is the position?

    d. What causes the bloody show?

25. What pertinent information can you gain from each of the following lab tests?

    CBC (Complete Blood Count)

    Hemoglobin

    Hematocrit

    VDRL (Venereal Disease Research Laboratories)

26. The obstetrician has ordered a "miniprep" and a Fleet's enema for Allison.

    a. Allison does not understand what a "prep" is. How will you explain it to her so that she can participate in an informed way?

    *b. What are three effects an enema may have on labor and birth?

    *c. If an enema is given, what safety factors should you consider when she is ready to expel her enema?

27. It is recommended that Allison receive only clear liquids or ice chips during labor. Explain the rationale for this.

*These questions are addressed at the end of Part I.

28. Choose a breathing technique commonly used in your area.

   a. Using it, give Allison a lesson in how to breathe during contractions.

   b. How will this vary during transition?

   c. Describe the technique you will teach Allison to use during the "bearing down" or "pushing" portion of the second stage.

   d. Now, select a friend and teach them the breathing pattern you chose. You might want to write out a description or draw the breathing pattern so you will be ready for your clinical experience.

29. What can you do to help Craig during the birth process? How can you assist him in supporting Allison? Describe support and comfort measures you can teach him or you yourself can provide if needed.

The physician has recommended fetal monitoring for a short time. After the reason for it is explained, Allison agrees to having a monitor placed on her.

30. Define the following terms used with fetal monitoring:

   a. Fetal baseline

   b. Fetal tachycardia

   c. Fetal bradycardia

   d. Baseline variability

   e. Early deceleration

   f. Late deceleration

   g. Variable deceleration

*31. Spell out the following abbreviations used in fetal monitoring:

EFM _____   UPI _____

FHR _____   HC _____

UA _____   CC _____

*32. The normal fetal heart rate is _____ to _____ bpm, short-term variability is _____, long-term

variability is _____ , and there are _____ decelerations.

*33. List five possible causes of fetal tachycardia.

a.

b.

c.

d.

e.

*34. List three possible causes of fetal bradycardia.

a.

b.

c.

*35. List three possible causes of changes in baseline variability.

a.

b.

c.

_____

*These questions are addressed at the end of Part I.

36. Explain the causes and the physiologic rationale for the following:

    a. Early deceleration

    b. Late deceleration

    c. Variable deceleration

*37. The electronic fetal monitor (EFM) uses a special graph paper to record the tracings for FHR and uterine contractions. The fetal heart rate is recorded in the upper half, and the scale numbered 30–240 is used to determine the FHR. The graph on the bottom is used to record a tracing of uterine contractions. The numbers on this section of the graph are not used unless the contractions are monitored with an intrauterine catheter. The graph paper is divided into small squares and when the paper moves through the machine at a rate of 3 cm of paper/minute, each small square equals 10 seconds. Note that darkened vertical lines occur every six squares. Therefore, the time interval between the vertical lines is 60 seconds, or 1 minute.

Using the above information, label the tracing represented in Figure 10–1.

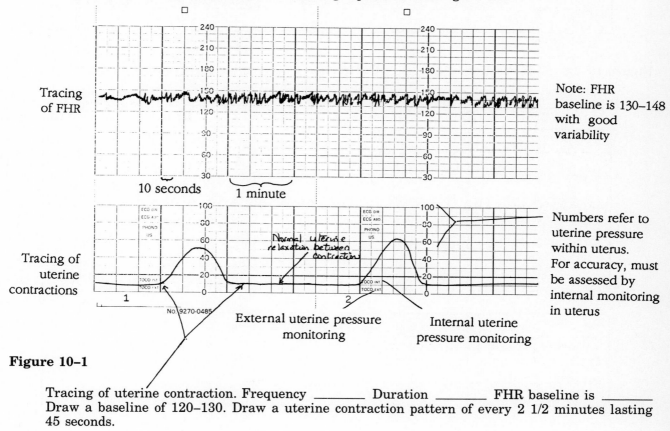

Figure 10–1

Tracing of uterine contraction. Frequency _____ Duration _____ FHR baseline is _____ Draw a baseline of 120–130. Draw a uterine contraction pattern of every 2 1/2 minutes lasting 45 seconds.

*38. Identify the steps to follow in assessing FHR and uterine contractions on a fetal monitoring strip.

---

*These questions are addressed at the end of Part I.

*39. Label the fetal monitoring strips shown in Figure 10–2.

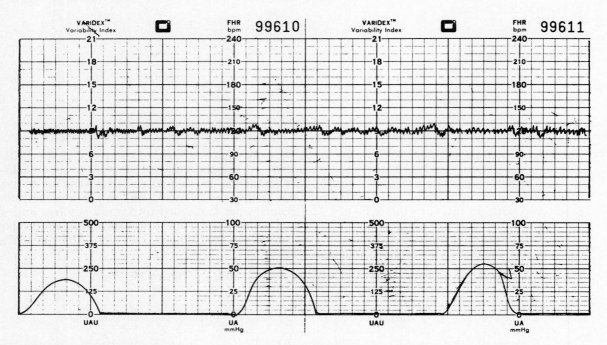

Figure 10–2A FHR baseline rate: _____ Contraction frequency _____ Contraction duration _____

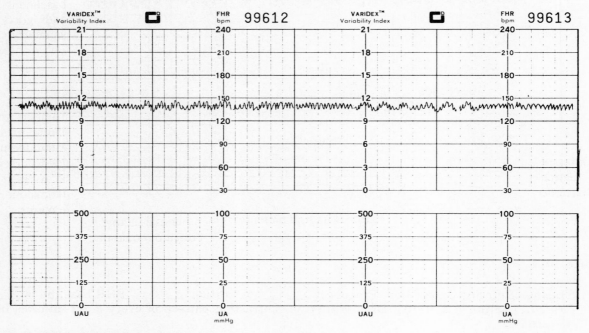

Figure 10–2B FHR baseline rate: _____

Check one of the following: normal rate _____ tachycardia _____ bradycardia _____

average variability _____ marked variability _____ minimal variability _____

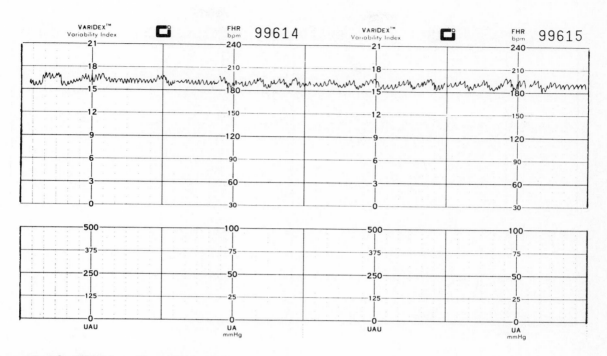

Figure 10–2C FHR baseline rate: _____

Check one of the following: normal rate _____ tachycardia _____ bradycardia _____

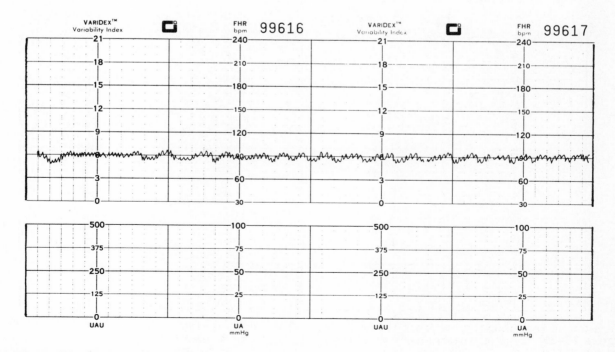

Figure 10–2D FHR baseline rate: _____

Check one of the following: normal rate _____ tachycardia _____ bradycardia _____

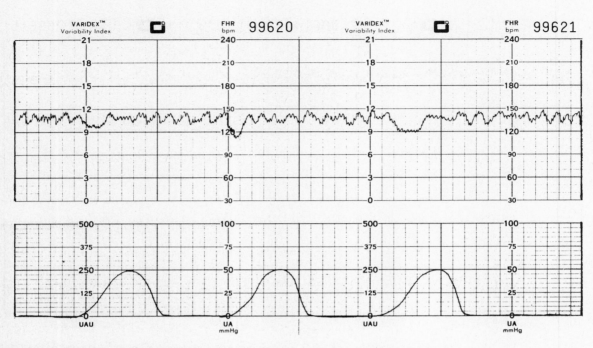

Figure 10–2E Type of pattern: early deceleration _____ late deceleration _____ variable deceleration _____ contraction frequency _____ contraction duration _____ Circle each deceleration.

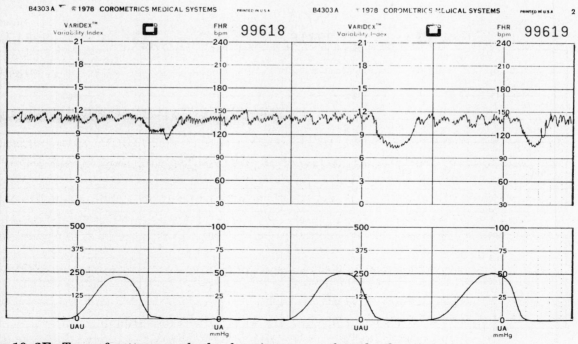

Figure 10–2F Type of pattern: early deceleration _____ late deceleration _____ variable deceleration _____

Variability: marked _____ average _____ minimal _____ contraction frequency _____ contraction duration _____

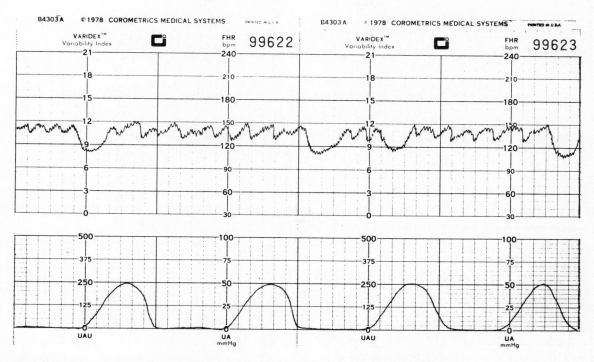

Figure 10–2G Type of pattern: early deceleration _____ late deceleration _____
variable deceleration _____ contraction frequency _____ contraction duration _____

40. Identify the immediate nursing actions and physiologic rationale for the following FHR problems:

FHR Problem	Nursing Actions	Physiologic Rationale
Late decelerations		
Variable decelerations		

41. The fetal heart rate assessment by EFM has indicated a normal pattern. At 5–6 cm dilatation, Allison asks for a pain medication. Stadol 1 mg IVP is ordered and is to be given by the RN in the birthing unit.

   a. Describe the assessments needed prior to administering the medication.

b. Describe assessments to be made after administering the medication.

c. List at least two indications that the medication is exerting the expected effect.

*42. As labor continues, you will use a Friedman graph to chart Allison's progress. Record the following information on Figure 10–3.

10 AM, 4 cm, −1
11 AM, 5 cm, −1
1 PM, 7 cm, 0
2 PM, 9 cm, +1
3 PM, almost complete, +2
4 PM, complete, +3

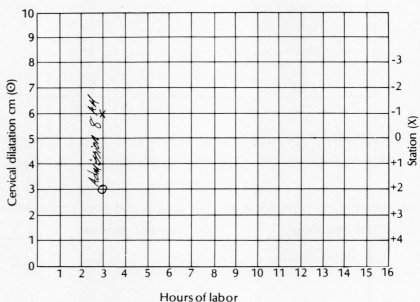

Figure 10–3 Sample Friedman graph. (Modified from Friedman E: An objective method of evaluating labor. *Hosp Practice* (July) 1970; 5:87)

43. Allison reaches 7 cm and becomes restless and impatient. What phase of labor is she in?

44. Allison begins to indicate many signs of discomfort and anxiety. Her previous methods to increase relaxation are no longer effective. Based on your assessment, you select the nursing diagnosis "Pain related to anxiety and difficulty maintaining relaxation." Identify at least four nursing interventions you think are important. Explain the physiologic rationale for each intervention.

    a. **Nursing Intervention**   **Physiologic Rationale**

    *b. Identify two anticipated outcomes or two signs that would indicate your interventions have been effective.

45. Allison complains of tingling and numbness in her hands and feet.

    *a. What is the cause?

    b. List nursing interventions to assist Allison.

    c. Identify findings that indicate your interventions have been effective.

---

*These questions are addressed at the end of Part I.

46. Allison reaches complete dilatation.

    a. Complete dilatation is _____ cm.

    b. What stage of labor is Allison in?

*47. List signs that indicate birth is imminent.

48. You prepare the birthing room for the birth. Describe the maternal positions that may be used during labor and birth. Identify the advantages and disadvantages of each and determine one situation in which you might suggest the use of that particular position.

49. How often will you assess blood pressure and FHR in the second stage?

50. Explain the support and comfort measures you or Craig can use to help Allison feel more comfortable as birth approaches.

*These questions are addressed at the end of Part I.

*51. The physician tells Allison that an episiotomy is needed. Describe indications for an episiotomy.

52. On Figure 10–4, draw a midline, left mediolateral, and right mediolateral episiotomy. Identify the areas involved with the following lacerations: first degree, second degree, third degree, and fourth degree.

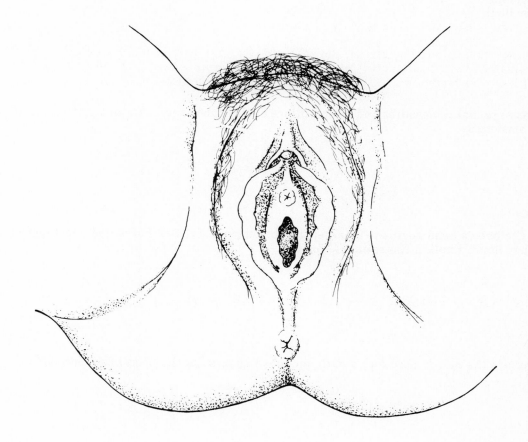

Figure 10–4

_____

*These questions are addressed at the end of Part I.

53. Complete the following chart regarding differences between a midline episiotomy and a mediolateral episiotomy.

Characteristic	Midline Episiotomy	Mediolateral Episiotomy
Indication		
Healing		
Discomfort after birth		

*54. Discuss prenatal measures and interventions during labor and birth that may decrease the need for an episiotomy.

55. As the baby's head begins to emerge, the obstetrician/certified nurse-midwife supports it with his or her hand. Explain the rationale for this.

56. Why are the baby's nose and mouth suctioned as soon as the head has emerged?

---

*These questions are addressed at the end of Part I.

57. A baby boy is born. Your first assessment of him provides the following information:

Heart rate 124

Respirations 24 and irregular

Flexion and movement of all extremities

Vigorous crying when suctioned with the bulb syringe

Pink body with some acrocyanosis

	0	1	2
Heart rate	Absent	Slow (below 100)	Above 100
Respiratory effort	Absent	Slow, irregular	Good crying
Muscle tone	Flaccid	Some flexion of extremities	Active motion
Reflex irritability	None	Grimace	Vigorous cry
Color	Pale, blue	Body pink, extremities blue	Completely pink

Figure 10–5   Sample Apgar scoring sheet. (Modified from Apgar V: The newborn [Apgar] scoring system: Reflection and advice. *Pediatr Clin N Am* [Aug] 1966; 13:645)

a. Record the above assessments on the Apgar scoring sheet (Figure 10–5).

*b. What is the total Apgar score? _____

c. Apgar scores are assessed at _____ minutes and _____ minutes following birth.

*58. The most crucial of the Apgar assessments are the heart rate and respiration. If the baby has a pink body, what do you know about the baby's heartbeat and respiration?

59. List the methods that may be used to provide warmth to the newborn in the birthing room.

60. Why should the newborn be dried thoroughly as soon after birth as possible?

*These questions are addressed at the end of Part I.

61. Allison places her newborn on her chest with skin-to-skin contact to maintain warmth. In some birth settings the newborn may be placed under a radiant heater. Explain how the radiant heater works.

62. As the nurse, you assess the number of vessels on the umbilical cord.

  a. Why is this important?

  b. How many vessels should there be?

  c. What problems may be associated with less vessels than expected?

*63. List two methods of assuring correct identification of the newborn after birth.

  a.

  b.

64. What positions may the baby be placed in to facilitate drainage of the respiratory tract?

65. What complication may result from vigorous, frequent oral suctioning?

*66. List the areas that will be checked during a brief physical assessment of the newborn in the first few minutes after birth.

*These questions are addressed at the end of Part I.

67. Describe ways you can facilitate bonding immediately after birth.

68. List specific maternal behaviors that would indicate Allison is beginning to establish bonding.

69. List four signs that indicate separation of the placenta.

    a.

    b.

    c.

    d.

70. Describe differences between a Shultze and a Duncan expulsion of the placenta.

    a. Method of separation from the uterine wall

    b. Appearance of placenta at the moment of exit from the vagina

71. Identify the complications that may be associated with a Duncan placenta.

*72. List three assessments of the expelled placenta that need to be made.

73. The obstetrician orders 10 units of Pitocin given intramuscularly after expulsion of the placenta.

    a. Explain the rationale for administration of an oxytocic medication following expulsion of the placenta.

    b. Identify the most important nursing interventions when administering Pitocin.

74. In the following chart, compare the oxytocic agents that may be used after birth.

Drug	Dose	Route	Effect on Uterus	Side Effects
Pitocin (oxytocin)				
Methergine (methylergonovine maleate)				

75. Explain the reason for assessing maternal blood pressure before administering an oxytocic medication following birth.

76. What blood pressure findings would indicate the need to delay oxytocin administration until consulting with the obstetrician/certified nurse-midwife?

---

*These questions are addressed at the end of Part I.

*77. You need to record the length of each stage on Allison's birth record, based on the following information:

        Contractions began at 0800
        Complete dilatation at 1600
        Delivered male infant at 1710
        Delivered placenta at 1725

    a. First stage _____

    b. Second stage _____

    c. Third stage _____

    d. Fourth stage _____

78. How does the length of each of Allison's stages compare with "norms" for primigravidas?

79. Allison begins her recovery period after birth. For each of the critical nursing assessments listed, indicate the expected normal findings.

Assessment	Frequency	Normal Findings
a. Blood pressure and pulse		
b. Uterine fundus		
–position		
–height		
–consistency		

*These questions are addressed at the end of Part I.

    c. Lochia

      –amount

      –color

      –presence of clots

    d. Perineum

      –episiotomy

      –lacerations

      –bruising

      –excessive swelling

      –hemorrhoids

    e. Bladder distention

80. Write a sample nurse's note that documents the expected findings at the first assessment after birth.

81. What is the significance of a boggy uterus? Describe the immediate action you would take if the uterus was boggy.

82. Allison complains of episiotomy discomfort. List some measures that may alleviate her discomfort.

*83. The recovery period usually extends for 1–2 hours after birth. List criteria that suggest normal recovery and indicate that the frequent assessments may cease.

*84. List the physiologic factors that contribute to discomfort in each stage of labor.

    a. First stage

    b. Second stage

    c. Third stage

85. How do each of the following factors influence the perception of pain in the laboring woman?

    a. Cultural background

    b. Fatigue

_____

*These questions are addressed at the end of Part I.

c. Anxiety

d. Previous experience

*86. The nurse completes pertinent assessments of the mother, the baby, and the labor prior to administering analgesics during labor. For each of the following, indicate findings that should be present prior to administration of the analgesic.

a. Maternal assessment

b. Fetal assessment

c. Labor assessment

87. Barbara Adams, gravida 1 para 0, is in the active phase of labor. Contractions are every 3 minutes, lasting 50 seconds, and are moderate. She is 7 cm dilated, 75% effaced, and at 0 station. Her membranes are intact, and the FHR is 140. With each contraction, Barbara cries out and thrashes in the bed. Her restlessness continues between contractions. She repeatedly changes positions and rolls her head from side to side. Her blood pressure and pulse rate have increased over the past 2 hours. The physician has ordered 75 mg of meperidine and 25 mg of promethazine, given intramuscularly when needed for pain.

a. In the above statement, circle all the findings that indicate it would be safe to administer the ordered medication. (Note: see answer to #86 to assist you if you are having difficulty.)

*b. Identify the three most important nursing considerations regarding administration of the medication.

*c. If all you have is a 100 mg/1 mL ampule of Demerol, how much will you draw up in your syringe?

d. Identify the landmarks you would use to administer the medication in the

dorsogluteal site _____

ventrogluteal site _____

*These questions are addressed at the end of Part I.

88. Complete the following chart on analgesic agents commonly used during labor.

Analgesic Agent	Dosage	Desired Effect	Nursing Actions	Side Effects (Maternal and Fetal)
a. Meperidine hydrochloride (Demerol)				
b. Butorphanol tartrate (Stadol)				
c. Promethazine (Phenergan)				
d. *				
e. *				

*Include any analgesics commonly used in your area.

*89. If Barbara continues to experience discomfort and needs additional pain relief, what types of regional anesthesia might be given?

   a. In active labor:

   b. In second stage labor:

90. Complete the following chart of the regional anesthetic blocks commonly used during labor or birth.

Regional Anesthetic Block	Uses	Nursing Implications	Side Effects (Maternal and Fetal)
Pudendal			
Epidural			
Spinal			

91. The following chart lists some side effects that may be encountered with the use of regional anesthetic agents. List the appropriate nursing actions for each side effect and explain the rationale.

Side Effect	Interventions	Rationale
Hypotension		
Decreased variability		
Uterine hypotonia		
Bladder distension		

*92. Action Sequence
You are the nurse in the birthing area. Carolyn Morse, a 25-year-old gravida 2 para 1 has been laboring for the past 6 hours. Suddenly you hear a low groan from her room, and then Carolyn begins to shout "the baby is coming." You rush to her room.

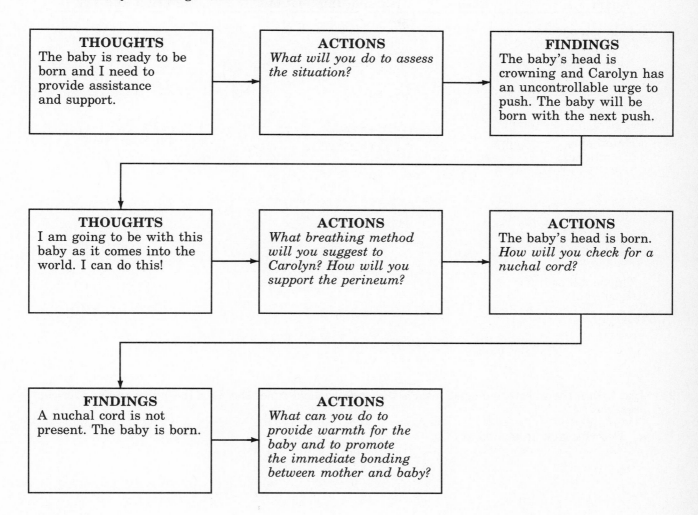

THOUGHTS
The baby is ready to be born and I need to provide assistance and support.

ACTIONS
What will you do to assess the situation?

FINDINGS
The baby's head is crowning and Carolyn has an uncontrollable urge to push. The baby will be born with the next push.

THOUGHTS
I am going to be with this baby as it comes into the world. I can do this!

ACTIONS
What breathing method will you suggest to Carolyn? How will you support the perineum?

ACTIONS
The baby's head is born. *How will you check for a nuchal cord?*

FINDINGS
A nuchal cord is not present. The baby is born.

ACTIONS
What can you do to provide warmth for the baby and to promote the immediate bonding between mother and baby?

93. General anesthesia may be used in emergency cesarean birth. Nurses must therefore be familiar with commonly used anesthetic agents. Complete the following chart:

Anesthetic Agent	Uses	Nursing Implications	Side Effects (Maternal and Fetal)
Inhalation agents			
Nitrous oxide			
Halothane (Fluothane)			
Intravenous anesthetic agent			
Thiopental sodium (Pentothal)			

94. Just before the anesthesiologist inserts the endotracheal tube, she asks the nurse to apply cricoid pressure.

a. Describe how this is done.

b. Why is cricoid pressure necessary?

c. Why is the pregnant woman at increased risk for aspiration?

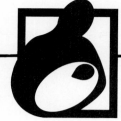

It's Your Turn

Describe the first birth that you were able to attend as a student nurse. What support measures were used? Did the expectant woman have a support person? How was the newborn welcomed into the world by those present? What were your feelings?

_____

_____

_____

_____

_____

_____

_____

_____

_____

_____

_____

_____

_____

_____

_____

_____

_____

_____

_____

_____

Selected Answers

This section addresses the asterisked questions found in this chapter.

3. There are four pertinent assessments of uterine contractions: intensity, frequency, duration, and the patient's response to the contractions.

7.
Contraction Begins		Contraction Ends	
0500:00		0500:40	(duration 40 seconds)
0505:00	(frequency 5 min)	0505:40	(duration 40 seconds)
0508:00	(frequency 3 min)	0508:45	(duration 45 seconds)
0511:00	(frequency 3 min)	0511:45	(duration 45 seconds)

   Remember, frequency is the time from the beginning of one contraction to the beginning of the next contraction. The frequency indicated by the first two contractions is 5 minutes; the frequency from the second through the fourth contraction is 3 minutes. This would be recorded as every 3–5 minutes. The duration is 40–45 seconds.

9. c. It is best to listen for at least 30 seconds and every so often you should listen for 60 seconds. During the labor, it is important to listen through a contraction to detect any slowing of the heart rate if an electronic fetal monitor is not being used.

   Guidelines for when to listen are as follows: every 30 minutes during the first stage, every 5 minutes during the second stage. It is important to listen to FHR immediately after the rupture of amniotic membranes, if the amniotic fluid has a greenish color (meconium staining), after an enema if given, after any analgesic or regional block, and with any significant change of maternal vital signs or change in fetal activity.

10. The woman should be lying on her back with a small pillow under her head. The knees are drawn up, with feet flat on the bed to increase relaxation of the abdominal muscles.

11. The fetal presentation is cephalic, and the fetal position is right occiput. Note, you were not given enough specific information to determine if the right (R) occiput (O) was anterior (ROA) or posterior (ROP). Think through what your hands would feel if the fetus was LOA, LOP, or RSA (right sacrum anterior).

13. The membrane status is ascertained beforehand because the lubricant used for the vaginal examination can change the reactivity of the Nitrazine test tape and thereby give a false reading.

16. Most sources recommend that the birth occur within 24 hours after rupture of membranes because after that time the incidence of infection increases. You will need to know when they rupture to be able to keep track of the 24 hours.

20. This is an excellent opportunity to gain additional experience as a patient advocate. Your response might be something like: "Mrs X would prefer not to have an amniotomy done."

21. You might say, "Mrs X has said she would prefer not to have an amniotomy. Is there something you are finding that she needs to know to reconsider her decision?" You are in a position to continue to be the client advocate. As you ask further questions, be direct and work to facilitate the exchange of information between Mrs X and her physician.

22. a. The membranes are intact. The Nitrazine test is negative.
    b. The most likely source of the clear fluid is the bladder.

23. a. A number of assessments are made while performing a vaginal examination. You can determine cervical effacement and dilatation; determine fetal descent, station, position, and presentation; and assess pelvic measurements.

24. a. 3 cm. If you did not answer this correctly, refer to a cervical dilatation guide in your textbook.

    b. Cephalic. The head feels firm compared to the softer tissues of its buttocks when the fetus is in a breech presentation.

    c. Left occiput anterior (LOA). The triangular shape is the posterior fontanelle. If it is felt in the upper portion of the cervix, the fetus is LOA. Refer to Figure 9–5 (or your textbook) for help in visualizing this fetal position. If you get this question correct, then you have a good understanding of fetal position.

26. b. Three effects of an enema are to cleanse the lower bowel, to stimulate uterine contractions, and to avoid patient embarrassment during the second stage of labor.

    c. If her membranes have ruptured, she should expel her enema into a bedpan. Consider leaving the siderails up to provide something for her to hold on to. If her labor is advancing rapidly, you will need to assess her labor status frequently. And when she is expelling an enema in the bathroom, she will need to know how to call for assistance.

31. EFM = electronic fetal monitor, FHR = fetal heart rate, UA = uterine activity, UPI = uteroplacental insufficiency, HC = head compression, CC = cord compression

32. The normal fetal heart rate is 120 to 140 bpm, short-term variability is present, long-term variability is average, and there are no decelerations.

33. The possible causes of fetal tachycardia include
    a. prematurity.
    b. mild or chronic fetal hypoxia.
    c. fetal infection.
    d. frequent repetitive fetal movements.
    e. maternal anxiety.
    f. maternal drugs.
    g. high maternal temperature.
    h. fetal arrhythmias (this is uncommon).

34. The possible causes of fetal bradycardia include
    a. fetal hypoxia.
    b. sudden hypoxemia.
    c. arrhythmia, such as congenital heart block.
    d. hypothermia.
    e. drugs, such as beta-adrenergic blocking agents (anesthetic agent used for paracervical block).

35. The possible causes of changes in baseline variability include
    a. maternal medications.
    b. fetal rest.
    c. gestation of less than 32 weeks.
    d. fetal hypoxia and acidosis.
    e. fetal malformation.

37. FHR baseline for the 6 min 40 sec shown is 130–148. The uterine contractions are every 3 minutes (frequency) with a duration of 60 seconds.

38. When assessing the fetal monitor strip, it is important to first evaluate and determine the baseline FHR. The variability is the next area assessed. The FHR is assessed for the presence of accelerations with fetal movement, which is a sign of fetal well-being. The FHR baseline is also assessed for the presence of decelerations. If decelerations are noted, they must be assessed with the uterine contraction tracing to determine if the deceleration is early, late, or variable.

39. The fetal monitoring strips depict
    a. FHR baseline of 120; contraction frequency every 3 min; contraction duration 60 sec.
    b. FHR baseline of 140 (136–146); normal rate; average variability.
    c. FHR rate 185–195; fetal tachycardia.
    d. FHR rate 74–82; fetal bradycardia.
    e. early deceleration; contraction frequency every 2 min; contraction duration 60 sec.
    f. late deceleration; minimal variability; contraction frequency every 2–3 min; contraction duration 60 sec.
    g. variable deceleration; contraction frequency every 2 min; contraction duration 60 sec.

42. A filled-in version of Figure 10–3 follows.

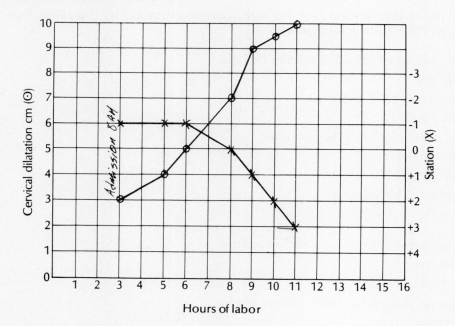

44. b. Anticipated outcomes may include: Allison cries out less during contractions, is able to doze between contractions, is able to maintain breathing during contractions, and remains relaxed during contractions.

45. a. The cause is hyperventilation, which leads to respiratory alkalosis.

47. The signs that indicate birth is imminent include a bulging perineum, increased bloody show, +3 station, gaping of the vagina, and an urge to push.

51. An episiotomy is done to prevent excessive stretching of the tissues and to prevent tearing or lacerations of the vaginal and perineal tissues.

54. During the pregnancy, some women prepare the perineum by doing exercises such as tailor sitting. The perineum may be lightly massaged with lotion or skin oil. During labor, the woman does not push until she feels a strong urge. The perineum may be massaged during this time to aid in slow distention.

57. b. The Apgar score is 8. One point off for respiratory effort and one point off for color.

58. A pink body indicates that the baby's heartbeat and respirations are in the normal range and the baby is probably not having difficulty. You could probably assume that the heart rate would be scored 2, and the respiratory effort would also meet the criteria for a score of 2. As long as the baby has not received any narcotics or medications that cause muscle relaxation, you could also assume that the baby will have a 2 on muscle tone and reflex irritability.

Overall, the heart rate and then respirations are the most important factors, because without them the other characteristics are not possible. Think about it: you cannot have a pink body and depressed or no respirations, and you certainly cannot have an absence of heartbeat.

63. Two methods of assuring correct identification of newborns after birth are
    a. application of name bands.
    b. Footprinting.

66. The brief physical assessment of the newborn should include
    a. overall size and general appearance.
    b. posture and movements.
    c. rate and irregularities of the apical pulse.
    d. respirations (rate, presence of retractions, grunting).
    If the newborn is stable, you may continue by assessing
    e. the head (general appearance, discoloration, fontanelles, flaring of nostrils, condition of palate).
    f. the neck (webbing or any limitation of movement).
    g. the abdomen (size, shape, contour, abnormal pulsations, number of vessels in umbilical cord).
    h. extremities (asymmetry, movement, number of digits).
    i. skin (discolorations, edema).
    j. elimination (record on newborn record any voiding or stools).

72. Assessment of the placenta should include
    a. examination of membranes: a missing section may indicate retention of a piece of membrane in the uterus, and vessels traversing the membranes may indicate placenta succenturiate.
    b. inspection of the umbilical cord for number of vessels, insertion site, and abnormalities, such as knots.
    c. inspection of the placenta for missing cotyledons, infarcts and/or areas of calcification, and overall size and weight.

77. a. First stage: 8 hours
    b. Second stage: 1 hour 10 minutes
    c. Third stage: 15 minutes
    d. Fourth stage: began at 5:25 PM and lasted until 7:25 or 9:25 PM (2–4 hours)
    If you missed this question, you need to review the definitions of each stage.

83. At the end of the recovery period the vital signs should be stable; the uterine fundus is in the midline, is firm, and is at the level of the umbilicus or 1–2 fingerbreadths (1–2 fb) below; the perineum is not excessively swollen or bruised; the episiotomy is not excessively swollen or bruised; and the skin edges

are well approximated. If the woman has had regional anesthesia, she has usually regained sensation in the affected parts.

In some places, the recovery period does not end until the new mother has voided.

84. a. First stage: hypoxia of uterine muscle cells during contractions, stretching of the lower uterine segment and cervix, dilatation of the cervix, and pressure on adjacent structures

   b. Second stage: hypoxia of contracting uterine muscle cells, distention of the vagina and perineum, and pressure on adjacent structures

   c. Third stage: uterine contractions and cervical dilatation as the placenta is expelled

86. Normal findings that indicate it is all right to proceed with administration of the analgesic are as follows:

Maternal assessment
- The woman is willing to receive medication.
- Vital signs are stable.

Fetal assessment
- The FHR is between 120 and 160 beats/minute, and no decelerations are present.
- The fetus exhibits normal movement.
- The fetus is at term.
- Meconium staining is not present.

Labor assessment
- Contraction pattern is well established.
- The cervix is dilated at least 5–6 cm in nulliparas and 3–4 cm in multiparas.
- The fetal presenting part is engaged.
- There is progressive descent of the fetal presenting part. No complications are present.

87. b. It is difficult to identify the three top nursing considerations that all nurses would agree on. However, we suggest that the top three would be: (1) assess the woman's history and present status to identify contraindications for administering analgesics, (2) determine that the woman is not hypotensive and fetal status is normal (FHR is in normal range with average variability and no variable or late decelerations), and (3) assure that the ordered medication is appropriate and the dosage is within the expected range. The next two nursing considerations would be: provide client safety after administration (e.g., ensure that side rails on bed are up, assist with all movement from bed, place call bell within reach) and reassess the woman and her fetus approximately 15 minutes after IM injection and 5 minutes after IV administration to assure normal effects and to identify quickly untoward effects. Were your top three within the top five that we selected?

   c. Formulas:

(1) $$\frac{\text{Have mg}}{\text{Have mL}} :: \frac{\text{Desired mg}}{\text{Desired mL}}$$

(2) $$\frac{\text{Desired}}{\text{Have}} \times 1 =$$

$$\frac{100 \text{ mg}}{1 \text{ mL}} :: \frac{75 \text{ mg}}{x \text{ mL}}$$

$$\frac{75 \text{ mg}}{100 \text{ mg}} \times 1 = 0.75 \text{ mL}$$

$$100 x = 75 \text{ mg}$$
$$x = 0.75 \text{ ml}$$

89. a. In active labor, the physician may administer a paracervical, epidural, or caudal block.

b. In the second stage, the physician may administer a saddle, caudal, pudendal, or local anesthetic.

92. *Action:* The immediate assessment should include looking at the perineum and performing a sterile vaginal examination if the head is not already visible.

Action: While placing your gloved hand on the perineum just under the vagina to provide support to the perineal tissues, ask Carolyn to push once more. As soon as the baby's head is born, ask Carolyn to pant. The panting will allow you a moment to suction the baby's mouth with a bulb syringe and to check quickly for a nuchal cord.

Action: You will slide your finger up along the side of the baby's head to feel for a loop of umbilical cord around the baby's neck. If you find a loop, bend your finger at the first digit (making a "hook") and gently slip the cord over the baby's head.

Action: You can quickly dry the baby with soft, warmed baby blankets and place the baby against the mother's chest and abdomen. Skin-to-skin contact provides wonderful warmth. You may also wrap the dried baby in another warmed blanket and place the baby on the mother's chest. The initial bonding process can be facilitated by providing time for the mother and baby together. Some mothers want to breast-feed their baby immediately after birth. You could assist Carolyn in breast-feeding if she desires.

Part II Self-Assessment

Do you know the following abbreviations?

Ab	HC
CC	LMP
EDB	Para
EFM	Rh
Dec	ROM
epis	VBAC
FHR	VDRL

Do you know the following words?

Duncan

Shultze

Add your own abbreviations or new words that you have learned:

Can you answer these questions?

The following multiple-choice questions will help you assess your knowledge of the content of this chapter. Select the best answer for each of the questions and then refer to the end of Part II to check your answers.

1. You are performing Leopold's maneuvers and determine that the fetus is ROA. Which of the following did you find?
   a. Round, firm object low in pelvis; small parts on mother's right side; and soft rounded shape in fundus
   b. Round, firm object low in pelvis; small parts on mother's left side; and soft rounded shape in fundus
   c. Soft rounded shape in lower pelvis; small parts on mother's right side; and firm, round object in fundus
   d. Soft rounded shape on mother's right side; firm rounded shape on mother's left side; and small parts at the level of the umbilicus

2. Which of the following describes contractions with a frequency of 3 minutes?
   a. A contraction that lasts for 3 minutes, followed by a period of relaxation
   b. Contractions that last for 60 seconds, with a 1-minute rest between contractions
   c. Contractions that last for 30 seconds, with a 2 1/2-minute rest between contractions
   d. Contractions that last for 45 seconds, with a 3-minute rest between contractions

3. You are palpating a uterine contraction and note that during acme the uterine wall cannot be indented with your fingertips. The intensity of the contraction is
   a. mild.
   b. moderate.
   c. intense.
   d. irregular.

4. You auscultate the FHR and determine a rate of 152. Which of the following actions is appropriate?
   a. Inform the mother that the rate is normal.
   b. Reassess the FHR in 5 minutes, because the rate is too high.
   c. Report the FHR to the physician immediately.
   d. Tell the mother that she is going to have a boy, because the heart rate is fast.

5. While performing a vaginal examination, you determine that the fetus is a cephalic presentation and that the occiput has reached the ischial spines. The station is
   a. −2.
   b. −1.
   c. 0.
   d. +1.

6. You note persistent early decelerations on a fetal monitoring strip. Based on your knowledge of this pattern, you would
   a. do nothing. The pattern is benign.
   b. perform a vaginal examination to assess dilatation and to determine whether the mother is ready to push.
   c. stay with the woman and observe what happens during the next contraction.
   d. turn the woman to her left side and start to administer oxygen by mask.

7. A laboring woman's membranes rupture suddenly at the end of a contraction. Your first nursing action would be to

   a. assess FHR.

   b. change the bed to enhance the woman's comfort.

   c. instruct the woman to push.

   d. notify the physician immediately.

8. Which of the following women would you expect to have the most rapid labor?

   a. Gravida 5 para 1 ab 3, at term

   b. Gravida 2 para 1, with breech presentation, at term

   c. Gravida 2 para 1, with left occiput posterior, at term

   d. Gravida 2 para 1, at 35 weeks' gestation

9. Which of the following would you normally expect if a primigravida with a breech presentation is in the transitional phase of labor?

   a. A decrease in maternal blood pressure

   b. An excessive amount of bloody show

   c. Severe back pain

   d. Slower progress than if the fetus was a vertex presentation

10. You would expect a cesarean birth for which of the following women?

    a. A gravida 2 para 1 who is dilated 6 cm after 3 hours of labor

    b. A primigravida who is dilated 6 cm after 8 hours of labor and is crying with contractions

    c. A primigravida whose pelvic measurements are diagonal conjugate 12.5 cm, biishial diameter 8.5 cm

    d. A primigravida whose fetal monitoring strip shows an FHR of 60 with contractions and who is dilated 5 cm

11. A multipara who has been in labor for 2 hours suddenly calls for the nurse and says "The baby is coming." After a quick assessment, you determine that the baby will be born with the next contraction. Which of the following interventions should be first?

    a. Call for assistance so the nursery can be notified.

    b. Instruct the woman to pant while you prepare to support the baby's head as it is born.

    c. Instruct the woman to push while you get a clean towel to place under her hips.

    d. Quickly return to the nurse's station to call for a physician.

12. Barbara, a 15-year-old primigravida, is in active labor. She has had no prenatal education. On admission, she asked numerous questions and seemed to become increasingly upset as you explained what the labor and birth would be like. As labor progresses, she becomes increasingly tense and is not tolerating labor well. You know her level of discomfort may increase further, because

    a. she is demonstrating marked anxiety.

    b. adolescents are usually unprepared for labor.

    c. adolescents have difficulty with authority figures.

    d. her labor will be prolonged.

13. For which of the following women would administration of analgesia seem most appropriate?

    a. 3 cm, with contractions every 4 to 5 minutes, lasting 30 seconds, and of mild intensity

    b. 5 cm, with contractions every 3 minutes, lasting 50 seconds, and of moderate to strong intensity; FHR 140 with good variability; patient relaxing well and breathing with contractions

   c. 7 cm, with contractions every 3 minutes, lasting 50 seconds, and of moderate to strong intensity; FHR 140 with minimal variability and occasional late deceleration

   d. 7 cm, with contractions every 3 minutes, lasting 50 seconds, and of moderate to strong intensity; FHR 140 with good variability; patient tense and unable to relax between contractions

14. The physician orders 75 mg of meperidine hydrochloride intramuscularly. You have on hand 100 mg in 2 mL. How much will you administer?

   a. 0.5 mL

   b. 1.0 mL

   c. 1.5 mL

   d. 1.75 mL

15. Which of the following observations would indicate a side effect of spinal anesthesia?

   a. Numbness of lower trunk and extremities

   b. Diuresis occurring on the second postpartal day

   c. Headache occurring on the first postpartal day

   d. Hypertension in the obstetric recovery room

Answers

1. b	2. c	3. c	4. a	5. c	6. a
7. a.	8. d	9. d	10. d	11. b	12. a
13. d	14. c	15. c			

Complications of the Intrapartal Period

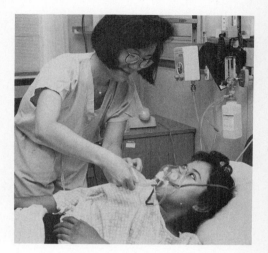

Introduction

As her pregnancy advances, each woman wonders about the course of her labor and birth. Relatively smooth labor and birth of a healthy baby are, of course, the desired outcome and are the result in the majority of cases. However, in some instances problems develop that complicate the process of birth and jeopardize the well-being of mother or baby or both. Early, accurate assessment of potential problems and appropriate therapeutic interventions are the key to achieving the best outcome possible.

This chapter focuses on the complications that may arise during labor and birth. Attention is given to the etiology and clinical picture in order to assist the nurse in assessment. Implications for both mother and fetus are also presented when appropriate. Anticipated interventions are then presented. Using this knowledge the nurse will be able to evaluate the effectiveness of nursing care.

This chapter corresponds to Chapters 25 and 26 in *Maternal-Newborn Nursing: A Family-Centered Approach*, 4th ed.

Part I Concepts, Critical Thinking, and Clinical Applications

1. Anxiety and fear may have untoward effects on the laboring woman and her baby.

   a. Explain the possible effects of increased anxiety and fear on the birth process.

   b. Describe the signs and symptoms you might observe when a woman is experiencing fear and anxiety.

   c. Identify at least one nursing intervention that would be important in decreasing a woman's anxiety and fear.

2. Draw a contraction pattern for hypertonic and hypotonic labor. Use different-colored pens so that the patterns will be contrasted.

3. Compare the effects of hypertonic and hypotonic labor on the woman and her baby.

*4. On the Friedman graph, draw a hypotonic labor pattern and a precipitous pattern.

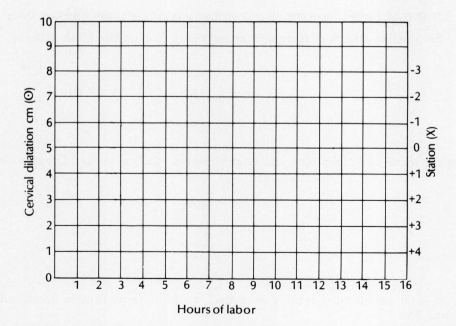

Figure 11-1 Sample Friedman graph. (Modified from Friedman E: An objective method of evaluating labor. *Hosp Prac* (July) 1970; 5:87)

---

*These questions are addressed at the end of Part I.

5. Discuss the medical treatment that may be suggested for subsequent births when a woman has had a precipitous labor and birth.

Postdate Pregnancy

6. Laura Collins, a 21-year-old primipara, is pregnant with her first child. Laura's last menstrual period (LMP) was September 8.

    a. Her expected date of birth (EDB) is:

    b. On what date would her pregnancy become postdate?

7. Laura does have a postdate pregnancy. Why will the fetus be at increased risk of having a variable deceleration pattern? What other problems may occur during labor and birth?

Occiput Posterior

8. Complete the following chart, which addresses four types of fetal malposition/malpresentations:

Fetal Malposition/ Malpresentation	Clues During Labor	Fetal and Maternal Implications	Neonatal Implications	Nursing Interventions	Medical Interventions
Occiput posterior position					
Face presentation					
Brow presentation					
Transverse lie					

9. Label each type of breech and the position of each on Figure 11–2.

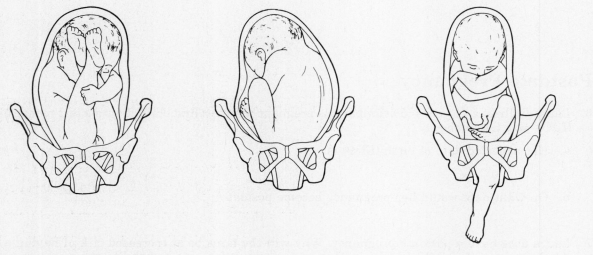

Figure 11–2

a. _____   b. _____   c. _____

10. Breech presentation carries an increased risk of prolapse of the umbilical cord. Draw a prolapsed cord in Figure 11–2C. Use a colored pen or pencil so it will stand out.

11. Prolapse of the cord causes pressure on the umbilical cord.

    a. Explain the fetal implications of a prolapsed cord.

    b. Describe what you would feel while performing a sterile vaginal exam.

c. On Figure 11–3, draw the type of deceleration pattern that may occur with prolapsed cord. First draw uterine contractions with a frequency of 3 minutes.

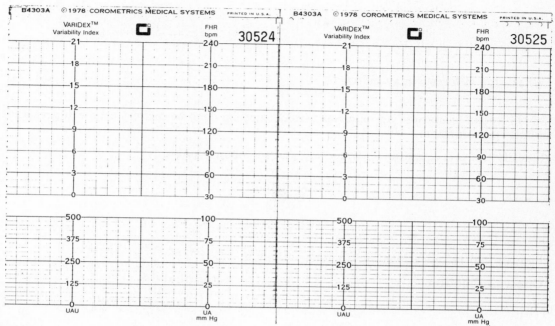

Figure 11–3

d. Explain why this type of deceleration pattern would occur.

12. List the complications that may be associated with breech presentation (excluding prolapsed cord; already addressed).

13. At term, most breech babies are born by cesarean. Explain the rationale for this. Include perinatal morbidity and mortality rates in your answer.

14. Sometimes a breech is born vaginally.

    a. Discuss the problems this may cause for the fetus.

    b. What type of forceps may be used?

15. At 36–38 weeks' gestation, an external version may be done to convert a breech presentation into a cephalic presentation.

    a. Identify the prerequisites for a version and include rationale.

    b. Identify contraindications and include rationale.

    Contraindication   **Rationale**

    c. Describe the version procedure with tocolytics.

    d. Discuss nursing interventions before, during, and after the version.

    e. Why would an Rh negative woman need to receive RhoGAM?

    f. Write out the pertinent points you need to cover in discharge teaching.

Multiple Pregnancy

16. Lisa Rote is in her second pregnancy. List two signs and symptoms that may indicate the presence of twins.

    a.

    b.

17. Identify three implications for Lisa of the multiple pregnancy.

    a.

    b.

    c.

18. Discuss the treatment that will be suggested for Lisa during her pregnancy.

*19. Discuss the implications of the multiple pregnancy for the fetuses during labor and birth.

*20. During labor, both fetuses will be monitored by electronic fetal monitoring. If one fetus begins to demonstrate problems with fetal heart rate (FHR), what will need to occur?

*21. List three signs and symptoms that would indicate fetal distress.

    a.

    b.

    c.

22. The major maternal complication that may occur following birth of twins is

    _____ . This occurs because _____ .

---

*These questions are addressed at the end of Part I.

Fetal Distress—Meconium-Stained Amniotic Fluid

*23. Meleah Stone, gravida 3 para 2, is admitted with contractions every 2 minutes, lasting 60 seconds and of strong intensity. Her membranes ruptured spontaneously 2 hours ago, and Meleah reports the fluid has been "greenish." She is breathing well with contractions and denies any discomfort. When assessing FHR, you located it above the umbilicus, at 140 beats per minute and regular. What would you suspect?

*24. Explain the possible reasons for the presence of greenish amniotic fluid. What special measures will need to be taken for the newborn immediately after birth due to the presence of the green-stained fluid?

Intrauterine Fetal Death

25. Anna Marinara, a 19-year-old primipara, calls the birthing unit and tells you she hasn't felt her baby move for two days.

   *a. When she arrives, you admit her and listen for the FHR. You don't hear anything with the ultrasound Doppler. She says "Did you hear my baby? Is she alive?" What will you say?

   b. What testing will you be able to anticipate for her?

26. Mr Marinara comes in after the tests have confirmed the death of their baby. Describe nursing measures you think will be important in providing support for him.

---

*These questions are addressed at the end of Part I.

27. Look at the resources in your community. What support groups would you be able to suggest in this situation?

28. Describe three nursing interventions that are important to include with the nursing diagnosis "Grieving related to loss of a child."

Placental Problems

29. Define *abruptio placentae*. What are the different types?

30. Define *placenta previa*. What are the different types?

31. Compare the differences and similarities between abruptio placentae and placenta previa.

	Abruptio Placentae			Placenta Previa	
	Marginal	Central	Complete	Marginal	Complete
Color					
Type of bleeding					
Amount of bleeding					
Pain					
Uterine contractions present					
Uterine relaxation between contractions					
FHR					
Incidence of disseminated intravascular coagulation (DIC)					

32. In the space below, write out your own situation of a woman with abruptio placentae and a woman with placenta previa. Include special unique details that will help you remember the characteristics of both conditions (e.g., the woman with a placenta previa could have a "P" in both her names and be wearing a bright red dress). Let your imagination go. The more bizarre the story, the easier it will be to remember.

33. Identify the primary methods of diagnosing abruptio placentae.

34. Identify the primary methods of diagnosing placenta previa.

35. Maria Thomas is admitted at 38 weeks' gestation with a marginal abruptio placentae.

    *a. Identify three of the highest priority nursing assessments.

    b. Your assessments reveal B/P 110/80; P 88; FHR 144 with average variability (data from continuous electronic monitor); uterine contractions every 3 minutes with a duration of 45 seconds, with almost complete relaxation between contractions; and dark vaginal bleeding.

    You analyze the data and determine two priority nursing diagnoses: one directed toward the potential for decreased cardiac output in the woman and one directed toward the potential for altered tissue perfusion in the fetus. Write these as nursing diagnostic statements.

    1.

    2.

    c. Identify one evaluative outcome that will indicate successful treatment.

---

*These questions are addressed at the end of Part I.

36. Dortha Haney, gravida 3 para 1, is admitted with moderate vaginal bleeding. She is at 39 weeks' gestation. She states that she is not having contractions but that she has had episodes of vaginal bleeding since the 20th week. An ultrasound reading demonstrated a marginal placenta previa. The FHR is 140. You know that a vaginal examination is usually done on admission to assess cervical dilatation. Will you do a vaginal examination now? Give the rationale for your answer.

37. Disseminated intravascular coagulation (DIC) is a potential complication of abruptio placentae and placenta previa.

    a. Why might this develop with abruptio?

    b. What other condition may it be associated with?

Problems with the Umbilical Cord and Other Placental Abnormalities

38. Problems may occur if the umbilical cord is longer or shorter than normal (18–22 inches).

    a. Describe problems associated with a long cord.

    *b. If a long cord becomes entangled, what type of FHR pattern would you see on the EFM tracing?

    *c. If a long cord has now encircled the fetal neck, it is called a _____ cord. What type of pattern would you see on the EFM tracing?

    *d. What problems may be associated with a short cord? When will you be most likely to observe problems in labor?

39. The umbilical cord is usually attached in the central portion of the placenta, but variations may occur.

    a. Draw a circle and place an "X" to demonstrate a battledore placenta.

_____

*These questions are addressed at the end of Part I.

b. Describe a vasa previa. What problems may occur in labor if this type of cord insertion is present?

Amniotic Fluid Embolism

40. Mrs Carey is a 28-year-old Gr 2 P 1 in active labor. She suddenly begins exhibiting signs and symptoms of amniotic fluid embolus. What will you be seeing?

41. a. You know that amniotic fluid embolus is more likely in particular situations. Write out a history for Mrs Carey that includes factors associated with amniotic fluid embolism.

    b. Describe the medical treatment that must be initiated immediately for Mrs Carey.

Hydramnios

42. Hydramnios occurs when there is more than _____ mL of amniotic fluid in the uterus.

43. Polly Brooks is diagnosed as having hydramnios. List three physical changes this may cause and identify at least two self-care measures you could suggest.

Physical Changes	Self-Care Measures
Severe lower back discomfort due to pronounced lordosis	Pelvic tilt: sit in straight-back chair, with feet elevated; wear flat shoes
a.	
b.	
c.	

44. Identify three fetal problems associated with hydramnios and a method of identifying each problem.

   a.

   b.

   c.

45. Describe the other conditions that hydramnios is most frequently associated with. Explain the rationale for the hydramnios with each condition.

46. When Polly's membranes rupture, she will be at increased risk for abruptio placentae. Explain the reason for this.

47. Polly's baby is born with esophageal atresia. Why is this more frequently seen in cases of hydramnios?

Oligohydramnios

48. Define *oligohydramnios*.

*49. The major maternal complication of oligohydramnios is _____ .

*50. Which fetal deceleration pattern are you more likely to see with oligohydramnios? Why?

51. Explain why oligohydramnios may be present when the fetus has a malformation or malfunction of the genitourinary system.

_____

*These questions are addressed at the end of Part I.

52. Describe the signs and symptoms the mother might notice with oligohydramnios.

53. Discuss the situation in which it would be more likely to develop.

*54. Some women have been told through "birth stories" that if you don't have enough amniotic fluid, you'll have a long, hard, painful, "dry" birth. If a woman asks you about this, what will you say?

55. Amnioinfusion is sometimes used to relieve the variable decelerations that occur when oligohydramnios is present. Describe the amnioinfusion procedure and explain the purpose.

Cephalopelvic Disproportion

56. Mrs Gonzales has a diagonal conjugate of 10 cm and converging side walls, and the fetal BPD (biparietal diameter) is 10 cm. What implications does this have for her labor and birth?

*57. What types of evaluation methods would you expect to be done when CPD (cephalopelvic disproportion) is suspected?

*These questions are addressed at the end of Part I.

58. Explain the rationale for a "trial of labor" for a woman with borderline pelvic measurements.

    a. What progress would you expect in cervical dilatation if the dilatation pattern remained within normal limits?

    b. What progress would you expect in fetal descent?

    c. In what instances would a cesarean need to be done?

    *d. Give an example in which the woman might need a cesarean for one birth and not for subsequent ones.

Induction of Labor

59. Describe the difference between indicated induction and elective induction.

60. List two indications for induction of labor. Explain why the induction may need to be done.

    a.

    b.

*These questions are addressed at the end of Part I.

61. Kate Morgan is scheduled for induction of labor. She is 40 weeks' gestation. Prior to induction, a CST is obtained and the results are positive.

   *a. Identify any contraindications present in the above example.

   b. List additional factors that contraindicate induction.

Table 11–1 Prelabor status evaluation scoring (Bishop) system				
	Assigned value			
Factor	0	1	2	3
Cervical dilatation	Closed	1–2 cm	3–4 cm	5 cm or more
Cervical effacement	0%–30%	40%–50%	60%–70%	80% or more
Fetal station	−3	−2	−1, 0	+1 or lower
Cervical consistency	Firm	Moderate	Soft	
Cervical position	Posterior	Midposition	Anterior	

Modified from Bishop EH: Pelvic scoring for elective induction. *Obstet Gynecol 1964;* 24:266.

62. Explain the Bishop score (see Table 11–1). What implications would the following scores have on anticipated induction success?

   a. Score of 3

   b. Score of 9

*63. Amanda White is admitted for an induction. She is gravida 2 para 1 and 42 weeks' gestation. Her membranes are intact. Amanda's obstetrician orders a continuous fetal monitor with a 15-minute baseline, followed by an intravenous induction of 10 units Pitocin in 1000 mL 5% dextrose in lactated Ringer's. The Pitocin is to be started at 1 mU (milliunit)/min by IV infusion pump. How many milliliters per hour will be needed to infuse 1 mU/min?

---

*These questions are addressed at the end of Part I.

64. Five percent dextrose in water is not routinely used for Pitocin induction because of the risk of water intoxication. Describe the signs of water intoxication.

*65. List the physical assessments and the findings that indicate Amanda's infusion rate can be advanced.

*66. List the problems that might occur in response to the Pitocin induction.

*67. After the induction has been in process for 2 hours, you palpate strong contractions and note the following information on the fetal monitoring strip (see Figure 11–4).

    a. FHR baseline is _____

    b. Variability is _____

    c. Contraction frequency is _____

    d. Contraction duration is _____

    e. Based on your assessment, should the IV Pitocin infusion rate be advanced?

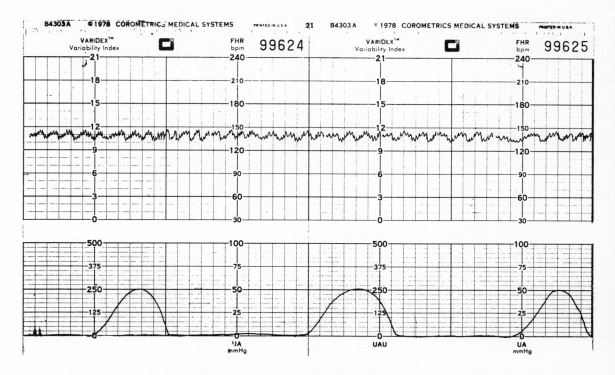

Figure 11–4 Fetal heart tracings. Paper speed 3 cm/minute; 6 small spaces equal 1 minute.

*These questions are addressed at the end of Part I.

*68. After an additional 1 hour of induction, you observe the fetal monitoring strip in Figure 11–5.

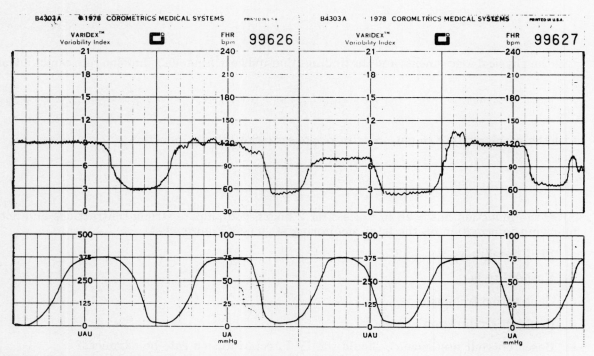

Figure 11–5 Fetal monitoring strip. 6 small spaces equal 1 minute.

a. What immediate nursing actions need to be taken?

b. What information from the strip did you use to determine your nursing actions?

*These questions are addressed at the end of Part I.

69. The obstetrician decides to rupture Amanda's membranes.

  a. Why might this be done?

  *b. What two assessments should be made immediately after the membranes are ruptured?

70. Explain the significance of the following characteristics of amniotic fluid:

  a. Greenish color

  b. Reddish color

  c. Foul odor

71. Intravenous Pitocin may be used for augmentation of labor. Explain the differences between induction of labor and augmentation of labor.

*72. Describe contraindications to augmentation.

73. Write out the dialogue you would use to explain the augmentation procedure to a laboring woman and her partner.

---

*These questions are addressed at the end of Part I.

74. If you note contraindications to the augmentation prior to beginning it, describe how you will communicate this information to the obstetrician.

Forceps-Assisted Birth

75. List three indications for the use of forceps to assist in vaginal birth.

    a.

    b.

    c.

76. Identify the criteria that should be met in order for the obstetrician to use forceps safely.

77. Define the following:

    a. Outlet forceps

    b. Low forceps

    c. Mid-forceps

78. Identify complications (maternal and fetal) that may be associated with forceps.

*79. Discuss the nursing interventions that are necessary during an outlet forceps-assisted birth. Include the teaching that should be done.

80. The new parents you worked with last evening during a forceps-assisted birth stop you in the hall today and ask why their baby's face is bruised and swollen on one side. They ask if it will go away. What will you tell them?

---

*These questions are addressed at the end of Part I.

81. A vacuum extractor may be used instead of forceps.

    a. Explain how this works.

    b. Why might the baby have a "chignon"?

    c. Describe the teaching that will be needed prior to its use. (Include maternal and fetal information.)

Cesarean Birth

82. Janel Thompson, a 24-year-old gravida 2 para 1, 30 weeks' gestation, is admitted to the birthing area for a repeat cesarean. Her primary (first) cesarean was done as an emergency measure when she began bleeding heavily from a complete placenta previa. The L/S ratio is 2.5:1.

    a. Describe how you will do the abdominal perineal prep.

    b. Describe the procedure for inserting an indwelling bladder catheter. What special implications does the low fetal head have on the insertion process?

    c. What teaching will you provide regarding the preoperative and postoperative course?

83. Janel's physician orders an IV. You insert an 18 gauge plastic cannula into the left forearm. The IV is to run at 150 cc/hr. The drop factor is 15 gtts/cc. You will set the drip rate at _____ gtts/min.

84. Describe the location of the incision in the uterus and advantages and disadvantages of the following types of cesarean procedures.

    a. Low segment transverse

    b. Classic

85. List the advantages of a low segment transverse uterine incision.

    a. Low segment transverse

    b. Classic

*86. Select the nursing diagnosis you think will be the highest priority for Janel's physiologic status in the recovery room. List at least two expected outcomes that you think are most pertinent for that diagnosis.

Nursing Diagnosis   **Expected Outcomes**

Janel will

Janel will

*87. As a part of Janel's preoperative nursing care, you identified "knowledge deficit related to postoperative course" as an important nursing diagnosis. You establish the nursing goal "Provide information regarding the expected postoperative course" and select appropriate nursing interventions to accomplish this goal. Describe objective data that will show your teaching has been effective.

*88. On her third postpartum day, Janel says to you, "I know that the cesarean was necessary and there was nothing that I did wrong but . . . Why do I feel like I failed somehow?" What will you say?

89. Describe the teaching you might do to help a father feel more comfortable during a cesarean birth.

Vaginal Birth After Cesarean Birth (VBAC)

90. Becky Saunders asks if she could have a vaginal birth next time even though she had a cesarean with her first birth.

    a. Which contraindications should be assessed?

*b. If she has a VBAC next time, she will be carefully assessed for which complications?

*91. Carla James, a 22-year-old gravida 2 para 1, had a cesarean birth last time. She has a vertical incision on her abdomen and asks "Does this mean that I can have a VBAC next time?" Select one answer.

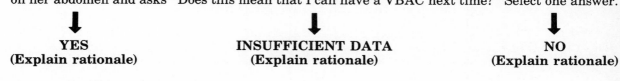

YES
(Explain rationale)   **INSUFFICIENT DATA**   **NO**
                                            (Explain rationale)   **(Explain rationale)**

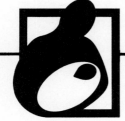

It's Your Turn

As you think about the clinical experiences you have had with child-bearing women who were experiencing problems, what one woman or couple stands out in your mind? What were your feelings during that time? What type of problem was it? What was done to help? How did the situation turn out? How did the experience change you?

_____

_____

_____

_____

_____

_____

_____

_____

_____

_____

Selected Answers

This section addresses the asterisked questions found in this chapter.

4.

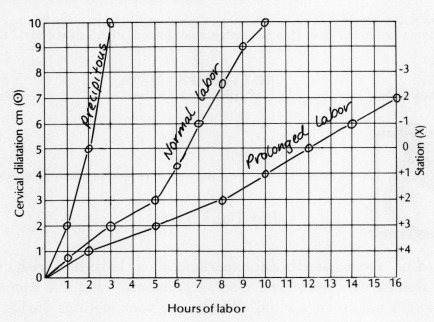

19. Implications for the fetuses may include
    a. inadequate nourishment of one fetus during gestation.
    b. premature labor, with associated problems of respiratory distress syndrome.
    c. difficulty in evaluating whether the second fetus can be delivered vaginally if the first fetus is delivered breech.
    d. interlocked fetuses.
    e. slow or interrupted labor because of overstretching of the uterus.

20. If one fetus exhibits problems, treatment must be initiated quickly in the same manner as it would if only one fetus was present.

21. Fetal distress would be indicated by any of the following:
    a. Loss of variability
    b. Severe late or variable decelerations
    c. Severe bradycardia
    d. Meconium staining in a vertex presentation
    e. Cessation of movement
    f. Hyperative fetal movement

23. You should suspect a breech presentation.

24. When the fetus is in a breech presentation, there may be a release of meconium due to the pressures occurring during contractions. In this instance, the release of meconium would most likely be viewed as physiologic. However, the possibility of fetal distress must be considered.

    When there is evidence of meconium staining of the amniotic fluid during labor, the birth team needs to be prepared to remove secretions from the newborn's naso-oropharynx immediately after birth. Suction is frequently used to remove these secretions. In the case of a breech presentation, the newborn will be suctioned as soon as the head is delivered. In vertex presentation, the naso-oropharynx is suctioned as soon as the head appears, and before the first breath is taken, so that the secretions are not drawn into the lungs with the first breath. The vocal cords will be visualized with a laryngoscope. If meconium is seen, suctioning will be done. Aspiration of meconium can result in meconium-aspiration pneumonia in the early neonatal period.

25. a. This is a very difficult situation. Anna deserves straight, honest information. You might say something like "I'm very sorry, Anna. I did not hear your baby's heartbeat. Your doctor is on the way. May I sit with you while we wait?"

    As a student, you may have fears that you will not hear the FHR and mistakenly think the baby is dead. In reality, you will be assessing FHR with your instructor or with birthing room staff. When you are just learning to listen to FHR and you either are not able to hear the FHR at all or are not sure what you are hearing, you might say to the nurse, "I'm not as experienced as you in listening to the FHR, and I'm not sure what I'm hearing. Would you listen to it now, please?"

35. a. The top three priority nursing assessments would be to assess maternal vital signs (B/P and pulse); auscultate FHR (or apply the EFM); and palpate the uterus to determine presence of contractions, irritability of the uterus, and relaxation between contractions.

38. b. Variable deceleration from cord compression.
    c. Nuccal; variable deceleration—the pattern may also progress into late deceleration and bradycardia with decreased variability.
    d. A short cord may not cause difficulty until the second stage when the descent of the fetus pulls on the cord. This may cause variable decelerations due to changes in blood flow. In some instances, abruptio placentae may occur.

49. The major maternal complication of oligohydramnios is dysfunctional labor.

50. As you remember, one of the functions of the amniotic fluid is to protect the umbilical cord from pressure. When there is a decreased amount of amniotic fluid, this protective function is lost. Pressure is exerted on the umbilical cord, and the cord is compressed. This will be demonstrated as variable decelerations on an EFM.

54. Amniotic fluid is produced all the time. When membranes rupture, the production of amniotic fluid continues.

57. The cervical dilatation and fetal descent will be carefully assessed by sterile vaginal examination. The fetal head will be evaluated for formation of a caput since (1) prolonged pressure on the cervix leads to the formation of a caput and (2) the formation of a caput will make it seem as if fetal descent is occurring. If slow progress persists, an x-ray pelvimetry will be done to provide actual measurements of the maternal pelvis and actual measurements of the fetal head to determine if CPD is present.

58. d. A cesarean birth may be required if a woman has an unusually large baby with one pregnancy. In subsequent pregnancies, if the baby is smaller, a cesarean birth may not be required.

61. a. Kate Morgan has a positive contraction stress, which means there are late decelerations of the FHR with contractions. The fetus may develop fetal distress and be compromised if contractions are stimulated.

63. The correct answer is 6 mL/hour. To compute this problem you need to start with the following facts:

1 mL Pitocin = 10 units

1 unit = 1000 mU (milliunits)

10 units = 10,000 mU

$$\frac{10{,}000 \text{ mU}}{1000 \text{ mL}} = \frac{x}{1 \text{ mL}}$$

$x = 10$ mU/mL of intravenous fluid

There are 60 minutes in an hour, and you want 1 mU/minute; 60 min × 1 mU/min = 60 mU/hr To obtain milliliters per hour:

$$\frac{10 \text{ mU}}{1 \text{ mL}} = \frac{60 \text{ mU}}{x \text{ mL}}$$

$10x = 60$
$x = 6$ mL/hr

Did you arrive at the correct answer? This problem requires a lot of thought, but it is important to be able to calculate Pitocin infusion rates so that the patient's safety can be maintained.

65. Immediately prior to increasing the rate of intravenous Pitocin infusion, you must assess the following:
    a. Maternal blood pressure and pulse
    b. Uterine contractions (frequency, duration, intensity)
    c. FHR (deviant patterns, variability)
    d. Fetal response (excessive activity)

66. The problems that might occur in response to a Pitocin induction include
    a. tetanic contractions.
    b. late or variable decelerations in FHR.
    c. a significant increase or decrease in maternal blood pressure or pulse.
    d. signs of water intoxication if an electrolyte-free solution is used.

67. The sample fetal monitoring strip provides the following information:
    a. The FHR baseline is 140 for the 8-minute segment. It is best to assess a 10-minute segment to accurately determine the baseline. If you caught this point, congratulations. You had to know the definition of an FHR baseline and correctly count the spaces to realize that only 8 minutes are depicted.
    b. The variability is moderate.
    c. The contraction frequency is every 3 minutes.
    d. The contraction duration is 60–75 seconds.
    e. No. The infusion rate should not be advanced because "good" contractions have been achieved.

68. The strip indicates severe problems.

   a. The immediate nursing actions would include discontinuing the Pitocin infusion and turning on the main intravenous line; turning the mother on her left side; starting oxygen administration at 6–10 L per minute; notifying the physician; anticipating preparations for effecting an immediate delivery.

   b. The strip showed severe late decelerations with minimal variability and tetanic contractions every 1 1/2 minutes lasting 80–90 seconds.

   If you were able to answer this question correctly, you have successfully correlated a lot of information. If you missed it, don't despair. Refer back to your textbook.

69. b. First, the FHR should be assessed immediately after the membranes have been ruptured. The rationale for this action is that the umbilical cord may wash down through the cervix as the amniotic fluid escapes. As pressure is exerted on the cord, the fetal blood supply may be compromised. Second, you need to assess the amniotic fluid for amount, color, and odor.

72. Augmentation would be contraindicated in the following instances: in the presence of fetal distress; with strong suggestions of CPD; with hypertonic uterine contraction pattern; in the presence of placenta previa; with multiple gestation. It is questionable with vaginal birth following cesarean birth.

79. The nursing interventions that are necessary during a low forceps assisted birth include the following:

   a. Explain the procedure to the woman and her support person.

   b. Encourage the woman to maintain her breathing pattern during application of the forceps. (Panting may help to relieve the "need to push" sensation that she will feel as the forceps are applied.)

   c. Monitor the FHR continuously.

   d. Monitor contractions. Inform the physician when a contraction begins and ends, because he or she will exert downward pressure on the forceps during a contraction.

   e. Provide support to the woman throughout the process.

   f. Ensure that adequate resuscitation equipment is available and in working order before the birth.

   g. After birth, assess the newborn for the Apgar score; facial bruising, swelling, abrasions, and/or paralysis; signs of cerebral trauma; and movement of arms (to detect paralysis).

86. Recovery from surgical anesthesia is a high priority for Janel. Nursing diagnoses directed toward this might be "Alteration in respiratory function related to shallow respirations" or "Ineffective airway clearance related to secretions in the respiratory tract." The second area of high priority is the discomfort that Janel will feel as she recovers from the anesthesia. A possible nursing diagnosis might be "Alteration in comfort related to pain from incision, surgical manipulation, and uterine contractions." You may think that other nursing diagnoses have priority; however, in the first hour or so after surgery, respiratory function and pain are essential areas to address.

87. If your teaching has been effective, Janel will understand the need to move her legs frequently during the recovery phase; she will take deep breaths and cough while splinting her abdomen with a pillow; she will ask for pain medication when she feels she needs it; she will cooperate with the turning and changing of position every 2 hours; and she will cooperate with ambulation to facilitate return of bowel motility.

88. As your mind races, searching for the "correct" response, remember that there are many ways to answer. Although you may be tempted to offer her reassurances that she is not a failure, this is a nontherapeutic approach. It will be helpful to focus on the "feeling" components that Janel seems to be expressing. Possible responses may be: "When the birth doesn't occur as you have planned, sometimes it feels like something is missing," or "When things don't happen as you plan, it feels as if something is wrong," or "It's hard to feel as if you've failed."

   Each of these possible responses focuses in on the feelings she may be expressing. It lets her know you have heard her and are willing to talk.

90. b. Rupture of the uterus.

91. Of the three choices, **Insufficient data** was the correct choice. The abdominal incision and the uterine incision do not necessarily match. The only way to validate the type of uterine incision is to review the surgical record of the first cesarean birth. If the uterine incision is a "classic" incision, a VBAC is usually contraindicated. If the type of uterine incision cannot be determined, many obstetricians would recommend a cesarean for any succeeding pregnancies.

Part II Self-Assessment Guide

Do you know these abbreviations?

BPD	ELF	pit
CPD	IUFD	TOL
DIC	MEC ST	VBAC

Do you know the following words?

hydramnios

oligohydramnios

Can you answer these questions?

The following multiple-choice questions will help you assess your knowledge of the content of this chapter. Select the best answer for each of the questions and then refer to the end of Part II to check your answers.

1. Signs and symptoms of the patient with hyperactive labor would include all of the following *except*
   a. contractions every 2 minutes, lasting 90 seconds.
   b. rapid progressive cervical dilatation.
   c. a prolonged active phase.
   d. discomfort that seems out of proportion to the uterine contractions.

2. A primigravida is admitted at term in early labor. You note on her prenatal record that her pelvic measurements are diagonal conjugate 10 cm, biischial diameter 7 cm. Based on this information, you would expect her labor to be
   a. within the normal length of time for primigravidas.
   b. prolonged, with slow fetal descent.
   c. prolonged, with failure of the fetal head to engage.
   d. "normal" through the first stage and prolonged pushing in the second stage.

3. In which of the following situations would it be possible to perform an outlet forceps–assisted birth?
   a. When the head is ballottable
   b. When the head reaches the perineal floor
   c. When the occiput is at the ischial spines
   d. When the biparietal diameter of the head reaches the pelvic inlet

4. The severe abdominal pain that may be associated with abruptio placentae is due to
   a. retroplacental collection of blood.
   b. precipitous labor.
   c. bleeding into the peritoneal cavity.
   d. marginal separation of the placenta.

5. A patient with partial placenta previa delivers following a 3-hour labor. The complication she is *most likely* to develop in the early postpartal period is
   a. hemorrhage.
   b. infection.
   c. hypofibrinogenemia.
   d. couvelaire uterus.

6. A 20-year-old primipara is admitted at term. She has a moderate amount of dark vaginal bleeding. Uterine contractions are every 3 minutes, lasting 40 seconds. The FHR is 140. Based on this information, you would know that
   a. you should suspect abruptio placentae.
   b. she is experiencing "normal" labor.
   c. she is near the end of the first stage.
   d. you should obtain an order for an analgesic.

7. A patient who has a breech presentation might have which of the following?
   a. A greater amount of bloody show during labor
   b. Slower labor progress than the norm
   c. More intense labor contractions
   d. A precipitous labor

8. While performing a vaginal examination, you note a glistening white cord protruding from the vagina. Your *first* nursing action would be to
   a. return to the nurse's station to place an emergency call to the physician.
   b. start administering oxygen by mask at 6–10 L per minute and assess the mother's vital signs.
   c. place a clean towel over the cord and wet it with a sterile normal saline solution.
   d. apply manual pressure to the presenting part and have the mother assume a knee-chest position.

9. You know that your initial nursing action for the situation in question 8 is effective when you find that
   a. the FHR is maintained at 140.
   b. there is no vaginal bleeding.
   c. the mother does not develop an infection.
   d. the mother's vital signs stay within a normal range.

Answers

1. c   2. c   3. b   4. a   5. a
6. a   7. b   8. d   9. a

Nursing Assessment and Needs and Care of the Newborn

12

Introduction

The extrauterine adaptation of the newborn infant is far more complex and exacting than previously recognized. The physiologic changes that occur are at once dramatic and yet subtle, requiring careful and continuous monitoring. Today's neonatal nurse assesses neonatal development, identifies common variations in each newborn, and recognizes abnormalities. The nurse assesses the newborn's changing status, develops nursing diagnoses, institutes interventions as needed, and evaluates their effectiveness.

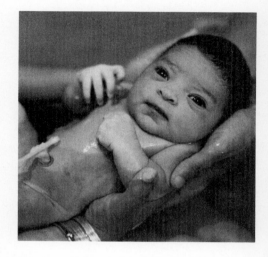

Parent education, a second major area of nursing responsibility, involves helping the family learn to care for its newest member. Inadequate parental understanding of the neonate's needs and requirements may jeopardize its health status and even its existence.

This chapter focuses on the normal physiologic changes that occur in the newborn. It then considers the assessments, nursing diagnoses, early nursing interventions, ongoing care needs including breast and bottle feeding, and health teaching required for successful function of the parent-infant unit. This chapter corresponds to Chapters 27, 28, 29, and 30 in *Maternal-Newborn Nursing: A Family-Centered Approach,* 4th ed.

Part I Concepts, Critical Thinking, and Clinical Applications

1. Describe four factors that are thought to stimulate the newborn to take its first breath.

   a.

   b.

   c.

   d.

*2. State four anatomic and physiologic changes that occur in the cardiovascular system during the transition from fetal to neonatal circulation.

a.

b.

c.

d.

3. Describe the changes in physiologic functioning that occur in the following systems during the neonatal period:

System	Neonatal Physiologic Adaptation
Hepatic	
Gastrointestinal Digestive enzymes	
Cardiac sphincter	
Lower bowel	
Renal Characteristics	
Specific gravity	
Urine output	
Immunologic	

4. List the normal values for the following areas of initial assessment of the neonate:

Assessment Area	Normal Values
Temperature	
Pulse	
Respirations	
Blood pressure	
Average weight of an infant in U.S.	
Average length	
Circumference of the head	
Circumference of the chest	

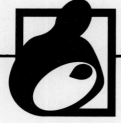

It's Your Turn

Do you remember the first time you held and cared for a newborn in your mother-baby rotation? How did you feel? What were your thoughts/impressions?

_____

_____

_____

_____

_____

_____

The following action sequence is designed to help you think through basic clinical problems. We've answered portions of it at the end of Part I.

*5. **Action Sequence**
   Glen, a 3450-gm baby boy, is born breech to Mrs Johns and has an Apgar score of 7 at 1 minute. Mrs Johns has requested to breast-feed Glen on the birthing bed.

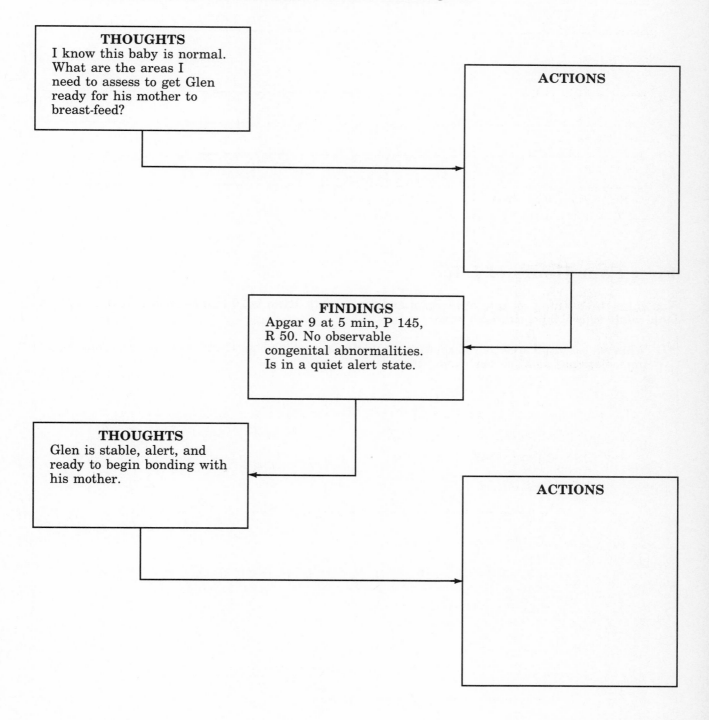

THOUGHTS
I know this baby is normal. What are the areas I need to assess to get Glen ready for his mother to breast-feed?

ACTIONS

FINDINGS
Apgar 9 at 5 min, P 145, R 50. No observable congenital abnormalities. Is in a quiet alert state.

THOUGHTS
Glen is stable, alert, and ready to begin bonding with his mother.

ACTIONS

*These questions are addressed at the end of Part I.

6. Write a sample newborn admission note.

_____

_____

_____

_____

_____

_____

_____

_____

First Four Hours of Life

You enter the birthing room to meet Ryan and his parents. Ryan is 20 min old and is in a quiet, alert state while interacting with his mother.

*7. What six essential areas of information would you ascertain about Ryan's perinatal, intranatal, and immediate postnatal period? Give your rationale.

a.

b.

c.

d.

e.

f.

---

*These questions are addressed at the end of Part I.

*8. List and prioritize six nursing actions you would carry out during the first 4 hours (transitional period) of the newborn's life.

   a.

   b.

   c.

   d.

   e.

   f.

9. Why are the newborn's hands and feet often cold?

10. Newborns can lose body heat through four mechanisms. Complete the following chart, stating the method of body heat loss and preventive measures that can be taken:

Loss of Body Heat	Preventive Measures
a.	
b.	
c.	
d.	

11. What position do most newborns usually assume? Why?

*These questions are addressed at the end of Part I.

12. On Figure 12–1, draw a series of numbered circles to indicate the correct sequence of auscultating a newborn's lungs. Place an "X" at the point where you should place your stethoscope in order to count the apical pulse.

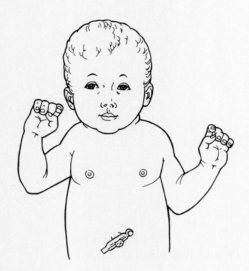

Figure 12–1 Auscultation of newborn's lungs and heart.

13. State four factors that influence the weight of a newborn.

a.

b.

c.

d.

14. Usual weight loss within the first 3–4 days of life for a full-term newborn is _____ %.

15. Why does the newborn commonly exhibit a "physiologic weight loss"?

16. Draw dotted lines on Figure 12–2 to show where you would measure a newborn's head and chest.

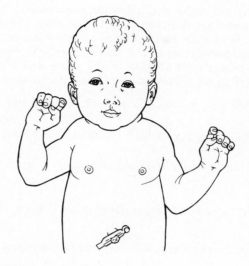

Figure 12–2 Measurement of newborn's head and chest.

17. What might a variation in the proportion of the head-to-chest circumferences indicate?

18. Describe how you would accurately and safely measure the newborn's length.

19. Why is a vitamin K medication given prophylactically to newborns?

20. What is the appropriate dosage for administration of vitamin K?

21. What is the preferred site for administering intramuscular injections to newborns?

22. Prophylactic eye ointments are instilled in the newborn's eyes in the immediate newborn period to prevent _____ , which is caused by _____ .

23. List two prophylactic eye ointments that are commonly used.

   a.

   b.

As part of the admission process, the newborn's gestational age is determined. Using Ballard's gestational-age scoring tool (Figure 12–3) determine Pam's gestational age.

Pam's gestational physical exam yields the following assessments of her physical maturity: her skin is cracking and has a pale area; some areas have no lanugo present; the breast bud is 1–2 mm with stippled areola; the ears are formed and firm with instant recoil; plantar creases extend over anterior two-thirds of sole; and the labia majora completely cover the minora and the clitoris. Assessment of Pam's neuro-muscular development shows posture with flexion of the arms and hips, 0 square window, 90–100 arm recoil, popliteal angle of 110, scarf sign with elbow at midline, and a score of 4 for the head-to-ear maneuver.

Pam's birth weight was 3202 gm, her length was 49 cm, and her head circumference was 33.5 cm.

*24. Pam's Ballard score is _____ , which equates to a gestational age of _____ weeks.

25. Based on the gestational age you determined, correlate it with Pam's weight and classify her as LGA, AGA, or SGA.

Plot Pam's length, weight, and head circumference on Figure 12–4.

*26. What factors might influence the neonate's gestational age score?

27. Why is it important to determine the gestational age of all newborns?

The normal newborn passes through specific periods of reactivity while making the transition to extra-uterine life.

28. Complete the following chart:

Period	Time of Onset	Neonatal Characteristics	Nursing Intervention
First period of reactivity			
First period of rest and sleep			
Second period of reactivity			

*29. While working in the nursery, you notice that baby Lewis, age 5 hours, has turned blue. Closer inspection reveals a large amount of frothy mucus in his mouth. What would be your nursing diagnosis in this situation?

---

*These questions are addressed at the end of Part I.

GESTATIONAL AGE ASSESSMENT (Ballard)

NAME _____   DATE/TIME OF BIRTH _____   BIRTH WEIGHT _____

HOSPITAL NO. _____   DATE/TIME OF EXAM _____   LENGTH _____

    AGE WHEN EXAMINED _____   HEAD CIRC. _____

RACE _____   SEX _____   EXAMINER _____

APGAR SCORE: 1 MINUTE _____ 5 MINUTES _____

NEUROMUSCULAR MATURITY

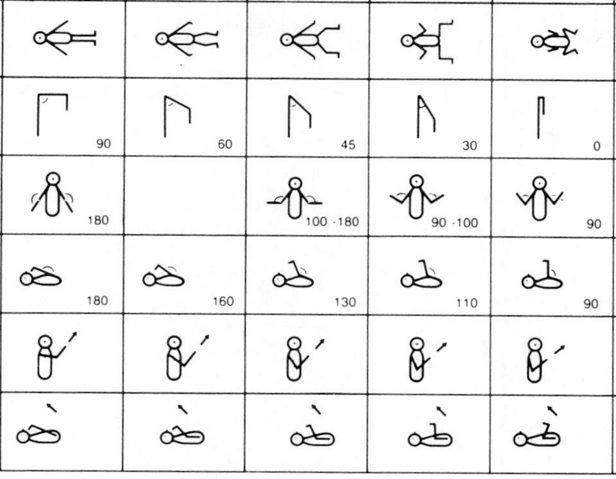

NEUROMUSCULAR MATURITY SIGN	SCORE 0	1	2	3	4	5	RECORD SCORE HERE
POSTURE							
SQUARE WINDOW (WRIST)	90	60	45	30	0		
ARM RECOIL	180		100-180	90-100	90		
POPLITEAL ANGLE	180	160	130	110	90	90	
SCARF SIGN							
HEEL TO EAR							

TOTAL NEUROMUSCULAR MATURITY SCORE

PHYSICAL MATURITY

PHYSICAL MATURITY SIGN	SCORE 0	1	2	3	4	5	RECORD SCORE HERE
SKIN	gelatinous red, transparent	smooth pink, visible veins	superficial peeling, & or rash few veins	cracking pale area rare veins	parchment deep cracking no vessels	leathery cracked wrinkled	
LANUGO	none	abundant	thinning	bald areas	mostly bald		
PLANTAR CREASES	no crease	faint red marks	anterior transverse crease only	creases ant. 2/3	creases cover entire sole		
BREAST	barely percept.	flat areola no bud	stippled areola, 1-2mm bud	raised areola, 3-4mm bud	full areola 5-10mm bud		
EAR	pinna flat, stays folded	sl. curved pinna; soft with slow recoil	well-curv. pinna; soft but ready recoil	formed & firm with instant recoil	thick cartilage ear stiff		
GENITALS (Male)	scrotum empty no rugae		testes descending, few rugae	testes down good rugae	testes pendulous deep rugae		
GENITALS (Female)	prominent clitoris & labia minora		majora & minora equally prominent	majora large, minora small	clitoris & minora completely covered		

Reference
Ballard JL, Novak KK, Driver M: A simplified score for assessment of fetal maturation of newly born infants. *J Pediatr* 95:769-774, 1979. Reprinted by permission of Dr Ballard and *Journal of Pediatrics*.

TOTAL PHYSICAL MATURITY SCORE

SCORE
Neuromuscular _____
Physical _____
Total _____

MATURITY RATING

TOTAL MATURITY SCORE	GESTATIONAL AGE (WEEKS)
5	26
10	28
15	30
20	32
25	34
30	36
35	38
40	40
45	42
50	44

GESTATIONAL AGE (weeks)
By dates _____
By ultrasound _____
By score _____

Figure 12-3

CLASSIFICATION OF NEWBORNS (BOTH SEXES) BY INTRAUTERINE GROWTH AND GESTATIONAL AGE[1,2]

NAME _____   DATE OF BIRTH _____   BIRTH WEIGHT _____

HOSPITAL NO. _____   DATE OF EXAM _____   LENGTH _____

RACE _____   SEX _____   HEAD CIRC. _____

GESTATIONAL AGE _____

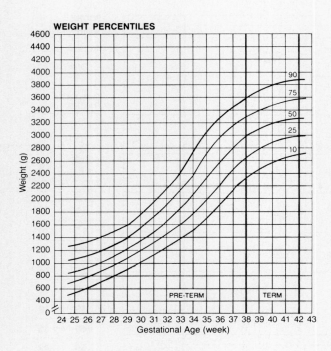

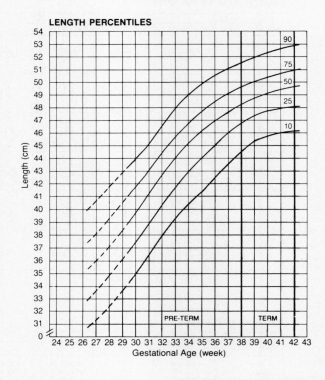

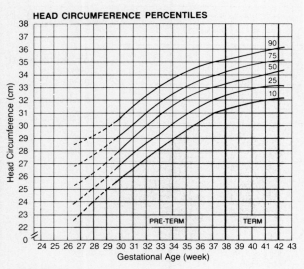

CLASSIFICATION OF INFANT*	Weight	Length	Head Circ.
Large for Gestational Age (LGA) (>90th percentile)			
Appropriate for Gestational Age (AGA) (10th to 90th percentile)			
Small for Gestational Age (SGA) (<10th percentile)			

*Place an "X" in the appropriate box (LGA, AGA or SGA) for weight, for length and for head circumference.

References
1. Battaglia FC, Lubchenco LO: A practical classification of newborn infants by weight and gestational age. J Pediatr 71:159-163, 1967.
2. Lubchenco LO, Hansman C, Boyd E: Intrauterine growth in length and head circumference as estimated from live births at gestational ages from 26 to 42 weeks. Pediatrics 37:403-408, 1966.

Reprinted by permission from Dr Battaglia, Dr Lubchenco, Journal of Pediatrics and Pediatrics.

Figure 12–4

*30.　Based on your nursing diagnosis, identify the immediate nursing interventions you would undertake.

At the end of the transitional period, or 4–6 hours after birth, baseline laboratory tests are completed.

31.　For each of the following laboratory values, identify the significance and appropriate nursing interventions:

Laboratory Value	Significance	Nursing Interventions
Central hematocrit of 68%		
Hemoglobin of 12.5 gm/dL		
Bilirubin of 15 mg/dL		
Heelstick glucose <45 mg%		

32.　As the newborn nurse, you would complete an initial physical assessment of each newborn. How would you proceed to do this physical assessment?

33.　Complete the physical assessment chart on pp. 258–263.

---

*These questions are addressed at the end of Part I.

Assessment Area	Normal Findings and Common Variations	Alteration and Significance	Nursing Response to Data Base
Posture At rest			
Awake			
Skin Color			
Texture			
Pigmentation			
Head Shape			
Sutures			
Fontanelles			
Shape/Size			

Assessment Area	Normal Findings and Common Variations	Alteration and Significance	Nursing Response to Data Base
Face			
Movement			
Eyes			
Placement			
Color and focus			
Movement			
Conjunctiva			
Ears			
Appearance			
Placement			

Assessment Area	Normal Findings and Common Variations	Alteration and Significance	Nursing Response to Data Base
Nose			
Patency			
Mouth			
Gums			
Palate (Hard & Soft)			
Tongue			
Neck Appearance			
Clavicles			

Assessment Area	Normal Findings and Common Variations	Alteration and Significance	Nursing Response to Data Base
Chest Shape			
Breast			
Heart			
PMI (Point of maximal intensity)			
Characteristics of pulse			
Lungs			
Characteristics of breathing			
Cry			

Assessment Area	Normal Findings and Common Variations	Alteration and Significance	Nursing Response to Data Base
Abdomen Shape and size			
Umbilical cord vessels			
Hips			
Extremities Position			
Shape			
Movement			
Genitalia Male			
Female			

Assessment Area	Normal Findings and Common Variations	Alteration and Significance	Nursing Response to Data Base
Spine 　General appearance			
Anus 　Placement			
Patency			
Neuromuscular 　Movement			
Tone			

34. Discuss the expected level of development of the following senses in the newborn:

Sense	Level of Development
Sight	
Hearing	
Touch	
Taste	
Smell	
Pain	

35. Identify methods that may be used to assess the newborn's vision and hearing.

36. Identify each of the following newborn skin variations, differentiating them by appearance, location, and significance:

    a. Harlequin color change

    b. Erythema neonatorum toxicum

    c. Telangiectatic nevi (stork bites)

    d. Nevus flammeus (port-wine stain)

    e. Mongolian spots

    f. Nevus vasculosus (strawberry mark)

37. Describe the dialogue you would use to teach a new mother about physiologic jaundice.

38. Why is the time of onset of jaundice important?

39. Compare cephalhematoma and caput succedaneum.

Characteristic	Caput Succedaneum	Cephalhematoma
Onset		
Location		
Composition		
Duration		

40. The newborn is born with various reflexes. Complete the following chart:

Reflex	Description	How Elicited	Age at Disappearance
Moro			
Tonic neck			
Rooting			
Grasp			
Stepping			
Other			

41. Identify four protective reflexes found in all normal newborns.

    a.

    b.

    c.

    d.

42. As you complete the newborn physical assessment, alteration in findings may be identified.

    A. Define each of the following:

       1. Hydrocephalus

       2. Cleft lip

       3. Omphalocele

       4. Myelomeningocele

       5. Polydactyly

    B. Describe the defining characteristics, physical alterations, and methods of assessment used for the following:

       1. Facial nerve palsy

       2. Cleft palate

       3. Hypospadias

       4. Clubfoot

       5. Congenital dislocated hip

Ryan has successfully progressed through the transitional period; he is now 6 hours old and continues to be adapting well to extrauterine life.

Daily Newborn Nursing Assessments

*43.   You are assigned to the mother-baby area. List seven daily assessments that are made of each newborn.

   a.

   b.

   c.

   d.

   e.

   f.

   g.

44.   Write a sample of a daily newborn nursing note.

   _____

   _____

   _____

   _____

   _____

   _____

   _____

   _____

_____

*These questions are addressed at the end of Part I.

*45. Helena Montoya wants to breast-feed Ryan. She tells you that she is really interested in breast-feeding but feels overwhelmed because she has so many questions and feels uncertain about beginning. She states, "I feel so full of questions that I wonder if I will ever know what to do." Based on your analysis of this data, formulate a nursing diagnosis that might apply.

46. Based on your diagnosis, what information would you give Helena about breast-feeding her son?

 a. Methods for encouraging the baby to nurse

 b. Positions for feeding

 c. Letdown reflex

 d. Breaking suction before removing the infant from the breast

 e. Length of time per breast

 f. Frequency of feeding

47. You stay and assist Helena with breast-feeding and answer her questions. Once she appears comfortable, you leave, but you check back with her periodically. Later in the morning when her baby is sleeping, you return to share information about other areas related to successful breast-feeding. What information would you share with Helena Montoya about the following areas?

 a. Nipple care

 b. Breast support

 c. Relief measures for breast engorgement

d. Maternal nutrition while breast-feeding

e. Environmental influences on successful breast-feeding

f. Use of medications while breast-feeding

g. Personal support systems

h. Available community resources

*48. Helena is only scheduled to remain on postpartum for one day. What actions can you take to help reinforce her learning so that things will go more smoothly when she is home?

*49. How will you evaluate the effectiveness of your teaching plan in meeting Helena's education need?

*50. How would you evaluate the adequacy of Ryan's fluid and nutritional intake while being breast-fed?

51. Ryan is 12 hours old, and he voids as you begin to change his diaper. What observations should you make about his voiding?

*These questions are addressed at the end of Part I.

52. You also note that Ryan's wet diaper has a pinkish rust color in the voided area. What is the cause of this?

53. If Ryan had failed to void within 24 hours after birth, describe the assessments you would carry out.

54. Within how many hours after birth would you expect Ryan to have his first stool and what would its appearance be?

55. When do transitional stools occur, and what are their characteristics?

56. Complete the following chart comparing the stools of breast-fed and formula-fed infants:

Characteristics of Stools	Breast-Fed	Formula-Fed
Frequency		
Color		
Consistency		
Odor		

Christy is a 2-day-old bottle-fed 3175 gm infant. Her mother is concerned because "she only takes 1 1/2 oz at each feeding."

57. What would your response be?

Christy is ready to be discharged at 3 days of age. She is now taking 2.5 oz at each feeding, approximately every 4 hours.

58. Her caloric/kg/day intake is _____ , and her fluid intake is _____ cc/kg/day.

59. Will this intake provide Christy with her average daily caloric and fluid requirements?

60. List at least five points to be included in a teaching plan to help Christy's mom successfully bottle-feed.

   a.

   b.

   c.

   d.

   e.

61. Christy's mother is concerned about the care of Christy's umbilical cord at home.

   a. What information would you give her about the expected changes in the umbilical cord from birth until the cord separates from the infant?

   b. What information about daily assessments and care of the cord do you want to provide Christy's mother?

   c. She asks, "When can I give Christy a bath?" How would you respond?

62. On your mother-baby unit, you are conducting mothers' classes on newborn characteristics. The mothers express concerns about the following common occurrences. How would you respond to each?

   a. "Can I hurt him by washing his hair over that soft spot? When will it close?"

   b. "All my family's eyes are brown, but her eyes are blue."

   c. "Why are there tiny white spots across the bridge of her nose and on her chin?"

   d. "Are my baby's eyes all right? There are bright red marks on the white part of his eyes."

   e. "He has white patches in his mouth. Is that milk? How can you determine the cause?"

   f. "My son's breasts are so swollen. Will the swelling go down?"

   g. "My baby is still losing weight. When will it stop?"

   h. "When I changed her diaper, there was blood on it."

   i. "Are her feet clubbed? They turn in."

j. "Why does his head look funny? The bones of his head cross over each other and look so narrow on the sides."

k. List other questions you have been asked by mothers and your response to them.

63. Mrs Smith, a gravida 3 para 3 who has a breech birth, unwraps her son's blanket for the first time to change his diaper. She suddenly puts on her call light. As you enter her room, she exclaims, "Look at his legs! They are up to his stomach and his buttock is bruised." How would you respond to her concern?

64. Prior to discharge, Ryan is circumcised.

a. What are your nursing responsibilities during and following the circumcision?

b. What home-care instructions would you provide?

65. Michael, a 3-day-old uncircumcised newborn, is ready for discharge. What instructions should you give his mother about penile care?

66. What type of immunity does the newborn receive from its mother?

67. List the nursing measures that are necessary to protect the newborn from infection in the birthing unit.

68. As newborn Michael is being readied for discharge, his mother mentions that her 3-year-old has just come home from preschool with measles.

   a. What information must you elicit from her in order to determine the significance for Michael?

   b. What health teaching is indicated for Michael's mother?

69. You are to present a newborn discharge teaching program.

   *a. List the essential components of this teaching program.

   b. How might you evaluate the effectiveness of your teaching?

70. Taking a new baby home brings changes within a family.

   a. What changes in life-style might they anticipate?

   b. What guidance can you give to help ease the baby into the family?

Selected Answers

This section addresses the asterisked questions found in this chapter.

2. The newborn's cardiovascular system accomplishes the following anatomic and physiologic alterations during the transition from fetal to neonatal circulation:
   a. Increase in aortic pressure and decrease in venous pressure as a result of loss of the placenta
   b. Increased systemic pressure and decreased pulmonary artery pressure due to decreased pulmonary circulatory resistance and vasodilatation
   c. Closure of the ductus venosus and foramen ovale
   d. Closure of the ductus arteriosis, which increases blood flow in the pulmonary vascular tree

   If you have identified these alterations, you have increased your understanding of what is necessary for the neonate to function as a new, independent individual.

5. *Actions:* Immediately after Glen's birth, you would dry him off, assess the heart and respiratory rates, determine the 1 and 5 minute Apgar scores, and then do a quick physical assessment for congenital anomalies.

   Actions: Place Glen skin to skin with his mother. Cover them both with a warm blanket to assist in maintaining his temperature. Assist Glen to suckle at the breast, and provide any support Glen and his mom may need to facilitate the bonding process.

7. As the newborn nurse, you should ascertain the following essential areas of information from the birthing room nurse:

   a. Previously identified perinatal risk factors

   b. Problems occurring during labor and birth, such as signs of fetal distress or maternal problems (abruptio placentae, preeclampsia, and prolapse of the cord all of which compromise the fetus in utero)

   c. Medications given to the mother during labor or given to the neonate in the immediate postbirth period

   d. The baby's Apgar scores

   e. Resuscitative measures administered to the newborn

   f. Elimination during the postbirth period (did the neonate void or pass meconium in the birthing room?)

   g. General condition and activity level

   If you identified these areas, you have a basis for identifying significant potential problems for the neonate. These areas of information provide a data base from which to make continued careful and significant observations and nursing diagnoses during the transitional period.

8. Nursing actions that you would perform initially and during the first 4 hours after birth would be

   a. assessing for any signs of neonatal distress.

   b. noting vital signs (including blood pressure in some agencies).

   c. measuring weight.

   d. measuring length.

   e. taking head and chest circumference measurements.

   f. administering prophylactic medications.

   g. scoring for gestational age.

   h. do blood work (Hct and heelstick glucose) at 4 hours of age.

   In addition, many institutions do a general head-to-toe admission physical. Other institutions may also do stomach aspirations, but this procedure is controversial and shouldn't be done until the newborn is stable because it can cause bradycardia and apnea.

24. Pam's Ballard score is 38, which equates to a gestational age of 39 weeks.

26. Factors that can influence a neonate's gestational age score are

   a. medications (especially on the assessment of the neurologic components).

   b. anoxia or hypoxia, which can result in decreased muscle tone and reflex determinations.

   c. timing of the scoring. For example, if sole creases are evaluated after 12 hours, the natural drying of the soles increases what appear to be sole creases; or if the labor and birth nurse thoroughly removes the vernix before the gestational score is determined, the score will be inaccurate.

   d. variations in the usual physical characteristics because of intrauterine conditions. For example, the infant of a diabetic mother and the premature large-for-gestational-age infant both have more breast tissue (increased subcutaneous tissue) than an infant of true gestational maturation.

   e. difficult birth, which may make determination of skull firmness difficult.

29. A possible nursing diagnosis would be "Ineffective airway clearance."

30. You would immediately aspirate the mouth and nasal pharynx with a bulb syringe, holding the neonate with its head down and neck extended to facilitate drainage as you aspirate the mucus.

   If you also recognize that there is an increase in mucus production during the second period of reactivity, you are well on your way to being alert and prepared to intervene in this very real problem.

43. Daily neonatal assessments should include
    a. vital signs.
    b. weight.
    c. overall color.
    d. stool pattern.
    e. voiding pattern.
    f. caloric and fluid intake.
    g. cord care.

45. The nursing diagnosis "Knowledge deficit related to breast-feeding correctly" might apply. Ms Montoya is obviously eager to be successful but has many unanswered questions. Her statement, even though not phrased as a request, was her way of reaching out and asking for assistance.

48. Because women are often discharged within 24 hours of delivery, it is difficult to effectively complete infant care teaching. You can help reinforce Ms Montoya's learning by presenting material in different ways (verbal instruction followed by practice, for example, or by showing a videotape followed by discussion). You can then reinforce positive behaviors. For example, if you observe Ms Montoya using the football hold, you might say, "I think it's really wise of you to try using the different feeding positions. Can you feel the difference in the suction when your baby is in this position?" When she is ready to leave, it is always helpful to provide handouts with specific information so the new mother will have a practical reference at home. By the same token, Ms Montoya may find it helpful to have the phone number of the mother-baby unit so she can call someone if questions arise.

49. Your teaching plan will have been effective if Ms Montoya is able to successfully breast-feed her infant and is able to demonstrate the techniques you have covered. For the cognitive content covered, you can ask Ms Montoya to describe to you the information you have shared. You can then discuss it briefly to learn whether she understands it fully.

50. The adequacy of the fluid and caloric intake of a breast-fed infant is determined by weighing him or her before and after nursing and by observing the quantity of urine and feces and their patterns of elimination.

69. a. Essential components of a newborn discharge teaching program would include the following:
    Bathing (skin, scalp, and nail care)
    Eye and ear care
    Nasal suctioning (use of a bulb syringe)
    Cord care
    Circumcision care or care of the uncircumcised male infant
    Care of female genitalia
    Diapering
    Positioning and handling
    Establishing a feeding schedule versus feeding on demand
    Burping
    Pumping the breasts and supplemental feeding for breast-fed infants
    Formula preparation
    Introduction to solids (what, when, why)
    Providing vitamin supplements
    Stooling and voiding patterns
    Sleep patterns

Continued

Clothing
Neonatal behavioral changes after discharge
Observation for signs of illness
Use of thermometer
Testing for phenylketonuria
Pediatric follow-up

Part II Self-Assessment Guide

Do you know these abbreviations?

AC   BAT   CC

HC   PKU

Add your own abbreviations or new words you have learned:

Can you answer these questions?

The following multiple-choice questions will help you assess your knowledge of the content of this chapter. Select the best answer for each of the questions and then refer to the end of Part II to check your answers.

1. The normal breathing pattern for a full-term infant is predominantly
   a. abdominal with synchronous chest movements.
   b. chest breathing with nasal flaring.
   c. diaphragmatic with chest lag.
   d. shallow and irregular respirations.

2. The average apical pulse range of a full-term, quiet, awake newborn is
   a. 80–100 beats per minute.
   b. 100–120 beats per minute.
   c. 120–140 beats per minute.
   d. 150–180 beats per minute.

3. Robert Scott is brought to the nursery by his father and the labor and birth nurse. He weighs 8 lb and is 21 inches long. You would tell his father that he is
   a. above the average weight and above the average length.
   b. below the average weight and below the average length.
   c. the average weight and above the average length.
   d. the average weight and length.

4. In the first few days of life, Robert's blood tests should reveal hemoglobin and hematocrit values
   a. consistent with active fetal erythropoiesis.
   b. consistent with high-O_2 fetal oxygen saturation.
   c. demonstrating shift of fluid to the intravascular compartment.
   d. lower than comparable adult values.

5. On the third day of life, a baby's glucose level is 40 mg/dL. The nurse should
   a. institute the nursery policy for a hypoglycemic infant.
   b. observe for clinical signs of hyperglycemia.
   c. recognize this as a normal value.
   d. substitute sterile water feedings instead of formula.

6. Vitamin K is administered in the immediate neonatal period because
   a. a newborn's liver is incapable of producing sufficient vitamin K to deal with transient neonatal coagulation problems.
   b. hemolysis of the fetal red blood cells increases coagulation problems.
   c. newborns are susceptible to avitaminosis.
   d. newborns lack intestinal bacteria with which to synthesize vitamin K.

7. While making rounds in the nursery, you see a 6-hour-old newborn gagging and turning bluish. You would first
   a. alert the physician.
   b. aspirate the oral and nasal pharynx.
   c. give oxygen by positive pressure.
   d. lower the infant's head and stimulate crying.

8. A 3-day-old newborn would be expected to have a fluid intake per feeding of
   a. 1/2–1 oz.
   b. 1 1/2–2 oz.
   c. 2–3 oz.
   d. 3–5 oz.

9. Newborns often regurgitate easily after feedings because
   a. control of their cardiac sphincter is immature.
   b. control of their pyloric sphincter is immature.
   c. peristalsis is reversed in their esophagus.
   d. their stomach is small and easily overfills.

Carl and Rita Grange had Ashley, a 6 lb, 11 oz normal term baby girl, 8 hours ago. Although they have had visits with Ashley, the nurse plans a teaching visit to describe characteristics of the normal newborn and to answer questions the couple may have.

10. Rita asks about newborn weight loss. Normal neonatal weight loss after birth
    a. can be prevented with adequate nutritional intake.
    b. can range from 5% to 10% in healthy babies.
    c. occurs only in very large or premature babies.
    d. reflects a potentially harmful fluid imbalance.

11. Carl asks about the "funny blue color" of Ashley's hands and feet. The nurse explains that this is a common and temporary condition called

    a. acrocyanosis.

    b. erythema neonatorum.

    c. harlequin color.

    d. vernix caseosa.

12. A small port-wine stain is located and pointed out to the parents. Which of the following remarks by the parents would demonstrate no need for further explanation of this mark?

    a. "Even though it's permanent, at least it's not too visible."

    b. "I hope it goes away soon, so she isn't marked for life."

    c. "My grandmother told me not to drink during my pregnancy!"

    d. "The doctor must have pulled on her too hard."

13. Ashley's eyes were treated with Ilotycin opthalmic ointment after birth. The nurse explains that the purpose of this treatment is to

    a. destroy an infectious exudate caused by staphylococcus.

    b. destroy gonococcal organisms, potentially acquired from the birth canal.

    c. remove a potentially harmful film that normally covers the eyeball.

    d. remove vaginal mucus and dead tissue cells after birth.

14. In response to the parents' request, the nurse performs some of the maneuvers to demonstrate Ashley's neurologic status. Demonstrating the rooting reflex, the nurse explains that the purpose of rooting is

    a. an aid in feeding.

    b. an automatic defense against overstimulation.

    c. interactive.

    d. protective.

Questions 15–17 pertain to the following situation. Joyce Palmer, a 24-year-old gravida 1 para 1, gave birth to Bryan, an 8-lb full-term infant. She is nursing her infant. She had a midline episiotomy. It is her second postpartal day. As part of your daily postpartal care, you assess each of the following systems for signs that they are functioning normally.

15. The breasts should be

    a. engorged and not secreting any fluid.

    b. engorged and secreting colostrum.

    c. full and secreting colostrum.

    d. soft and secreting milk.

16. You are instructing Joyce about measures to help relieve her progressive breast discomfort. Which of the following would you suggest to her?

    a. Application of a firm breast binder to compress the breasts

    b. Application of a warm moist towel and an uplifting support binder or good support brassiere

    c. Application of ice packs to the breasts

    d. Decrease fluid intake and application of an uplifting support binder or good support brassiere

17. Which of the following instructions should you give to Joyce about breast care?
    a. Wash nipples before each feeding with a mild soap.
    b. Wash nipples daily with warm water and mild soap.
    c. Wash the nipples once a day with plain water.
    d. Wash your nipples with a mild antiseptic prior to each feeding.

18. Mrs Thomas, a gravida 1 para 1, is planning to bottle-feed Jennifer. She knows that Jennifer should be allowed to set her own schedule but she asks how often that will be. Infants need to have formula approximately how many times a day?
    a. Two to four
    b. Four to six
    c. Six to eight
    d. Eight to ten

Answers

1. a	2. c	3. d	4. a	5. a	6. d
7. b	8. c	9. a	10. b	11. a	12. a
13. b	14. a	15. a	16. b	17. c	18. c

Nursing Assessment and Care of Newborn at Risk

13

Introduction

The majority of pregnancies end with the birth of a healthy term infant who flourishes with appropriate parental care and support. However, some infants develop serious problems during their early hours and days of life. These infants are classified as "high risk" or "at risk." In many instances the maternal or fetal factors that increase risk can be predicted during the antepartal period. In other cases the infant's risk status results from insults or complications that occur during labor and birth. In both instances appropriate interventions can significantly improve the baby's outlook.

This chapter first considers the factors that contribute to the development of a high-risk infant and the commonly used methods of assessing an infant's status. It then focuses on many of the problems that may afflict high-risk infants, with emphasis on nursing assessments and interventions and, finally, on evaluation of the effectiveness of care. This chapter corresponds to Chapters 31 and 32 in *Maternal-Newborn Nursing: A Family-Centered Approach,* 4th ed.

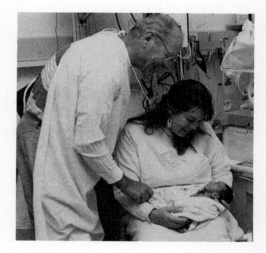

Part I Concepts, Critical Thinking, and Clinical Applications

1. Identify six maternal factors that may contribute to the birth of an at-risk infant.

   a.

   b.

   c.

   d.

   e.

   f.

Using a neonatal classification and mortality chart, plot each newborn's gestational age and weight and identify the appropriate classification for each of the following newborns (each newborn may belong to a classification group based on both gestational age and weight):

*2. Baby Joey is 36–37 weeks' gestation, twin B, weighing 1500 gm.

   Classification _____

3. Baby Gwynn is 42 1/2 weeks' gestation by clinical determination and weighs 3150 gm.

   Classification _____

---

*These questions are addressed at the end of Part I.

4. Baby Sara is 34 weeks and weighs 2060 gm.

   Classification _____

5. Baby Mark is a 39-week newborn weighing 3950 gm.

   Classification _____

6. Baby Carla is 41 weeks and weighs 2500 gm.

   Classification _____

SGA Infants

7. List four maternal causes for an SGA infant.

   a.

   b.

   c.

   d.

*8. What physical findings would you expect when scoring the gestational age of an SGA infant?

9. Based on the potential complications associated with an SGA newborn, formulate two nursing diagnoses that will guide your plan of care.

10. Describe the potential long-term implications for an SGA infant.

---

*These questions are addressed at the end of Part I.

Infant of a Diabetic Mother (IDM)

11. Richard is a 36 weeks' gestation newborn, weighing 9 lb, 1 oz. His admitting nursery information indicates that his mother is a class C diabetic. What physical characteristics would you expect him to have?

12. Identify the cause for Richard's large size.

13. What laboratory test should be carried out on Richard and when?

14. You would anticipate Richard's blood glucose at birth to be _____.

15. Richard may show beginning signs of hypoglycemia _____ hours after delivery.

16. Hypoglycemia occurs when blood glucose levels fall below _____ mg/dL.

17. What signs of developing hypoglycemia would you observe in Richard?

18. Identify the interventions you would carry out relative to the assessment and treatment of hypoglycemia.

19. Richard is susceptible to the following complications. State the cause and treatment of each.

Complication	Cause	Treatment
Birth trauma		
Respiratory distress		
Hyperbilirubinemia		

Postterm Infants

*20. List three obstetric indications of a postterm pregnancy.

    a.

    b.

    c.

21. Describe the clinical picture of a postterm infant.

22. Describe the potential long-term implications for a postterm infant.

---

*These questions are addressed at the end of Part I.

Preterm Infant

23. List four major causes of prematurity.

    a.

    b.

    c.

    d.

24. Describe five physical characteristics you would expect to find in an AGA 35-week gestational age newborn.

    a.

    b.

    c.

    d.

    e.

*25. You have just received a call from the birthing room that a preterm infant has been born. What preparations and equipment should you get ready in order to receive this infant?

*26. A preterm infant arrives in the nursery. What three initial assessments should you make?

    a.

    b.

    c.

27. The physical characteristics and immaturity of preterm infants' body systems cause them to exhibit a number of physiologic problems. For each of the following problems, identify the cause and the appropriate nursing interventions:

Physiologic Problem	Cause	Nursing Interventions
Temperature instability		
Respiratory distress		
Susceptibility to infection		
Adequate caloric and fluid intake		
Hypocalcemia		
Hypoglycemia		

Drug-Addicted Infants

28. Claire, a 2-day-old, 2000 gm neonate, is observed to be going through withdrawal. Her 18-year-old mother was addicted to heroin during the pregnancy. List six symptoms of withdrawal you may observe in Claire.

a.

b.

c.

d.

e.

f.

29. Describe five nursing interventions you may implement to help Claire through the withdrawal period.

    a.

    b.

    c.

    d.

    e.

Newborn with AIDS

30. What signs and symptoms may be seen in a newborn with AIDS?

31. How do the CDC's universal precautions apply to your nursing care of a newborn born to a woman suspected of having AIDS?

Immediate newborn care for all at–risk newborns, in addition to providing warmth, is centered around determination of the need for resuscitation and maintenance of a patent airway. For the newborns described below, state the resuscitative measures that you would initiate.

32. Baby Jean, a 31-week preterm newborn, was born vaginally to a 20-year-old woman who came to the ER in advanced active labor. Based on a quick assessment at the time of birth, Jean is given an Apgar of 4. What resuscitative measures should be instituted?

33. Baby Ken, a 43-1/2-week postterm newborn, experienced early deceleration in labor. Yellow-green amniotic fluid was present at the time of membrane rupture.

   a. Ken is at risk of what neonatal problem?

   b. What resuscitative measures should be instituted as soon as his head and face appear on the perineum?

   c. What additional resuscitative measures or actions do you anticipate will be carried out after Ken is delivered?

The following situation has been included to challenge your critical thinking. Read the situation and then answer the question "yes" or "no."

*34. Celeste, a 3200 gm term baby, is born vaginally. The amniotic fluid is lightly meconium stained. She was suctioned on the perineum and cried vigorously within 30 seconds of birth.

   Is Celeste a candidate for further resuscitation measures?

   _____
                    ⇓   ⇓

   Yes (Why? _____)   No (Why not? _____)
   Identify the therapy you would   Identify your most pressing
   expect to be initiated.   nursing goal.

---

*These questions are addressed at the end of Part I.

Brian, a term baby, was born vaginally 2 hours after his mother received 75 mg of Demerol IM. He has some flexion of extremities and acrocyanosis, HR-96, slow and irregular respiratory effort, and facial grimace. His Apgar at 1 min is 5. You are assisting the physician/neonatal nurse practitioner with the resuscitation.

35. Why is deep, vigorous suctioning of the airway to be avoided?

36. During bag-and-mask resuscitation you watch Brian's resuscitation bag to ensure it is inflating adequately and the pressure manometer to achieve the desired pressure of _____ cm H_2O at a rate of _____ times/min.

*37. Based on Brian's intrapartal history, what other resuscitative measures does he need?

38. Complete the chart on drugs used in newborn resuscitation.

Drug	Dose/Route	Indications	Nursing Considerations
Epinephrine			
Sodium bicarbonate			
Naloxone hydrochloride			
Dopamine			

Respiratory Distress Syndrome

Tricia, a 3-1/2 lb (1587 gm) neonate with a gestational age of 34 weeks, was born at 10:30 PM. Her Apgar score at 1 minute was 3, necessitating resuscitation via intubation and oxygen administration. On admission to the high-risk nursery, her vital signs are pulse 150, respirations 50, and rectal temperature of 96.2°F (35.7°C). She is placed in a radiant heat warmer, and an umbilical artery catheter is inserted for intravenous infusion.

*39. You are to assess Tricia for signs of respiratory distress. List six signs indicative of developing respiratory distress.

a.

b.

c.

d.

e.

f.

*40. Additional physical assessment data on Tricia's respiratory status reveals minimal nasal flaring, chest lag on inspiration with just visible intercostal (lower chest) and xiphoid retractions, and audible expiratory grunting. Using the Silverman-Andersen index (Figure 13–1), your respiratory distress score for Tricia would be _____ .

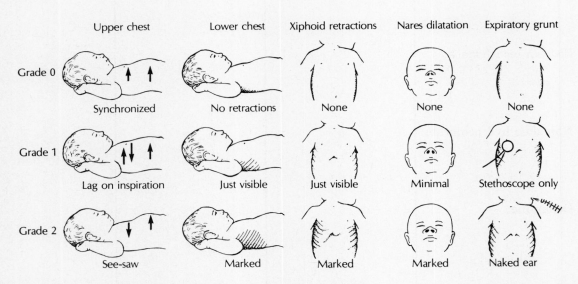

Figure 13–1 Evaluation of respiratory status using the Silverman-Andersen index. (From Ross Laboratories, Nursing Inservice Aid no. 2, Columbus, Ohio; and Silverman WA, Andersen DH: *Pediatrics* 1956; 17:1. Copyright © 1956: American Academy of Pediatrics)

---

*These questions are addressed at the end of Part I.

*41. What is the significance of Tricia's Silverman-Andersen score?

*42. What three factors may predispose Tricia to develop respiratory distress syndrome?

   a.

   b.

   c.

43. It is now 2 AM, and Tricia is showing signs of respiratory distress syndrome. She is placed in an oxygen hood with a warmed, humidified oxygen concentration of 70%. What is the rationale for administering warmed and humidified oxygen?

44. Tricia's respirations are now 65 per minute; she has an apical pulse of 152–176 beats per minute; and her arterial blood gases show a pH of 7.3, PO_2 of 55 mm Hg, and PCO_2 of 69 mm Hg.

   *a. What are your nursing responsibilities during oxygen administration?

   b. How would you evaluate the effectiveness of Tricia's oxygen therapy?

---

*These questions are addressed at the end of Part I.

45. Oxygen administration to the premature infant can lead to complications. Briefly discuss the pathology and nursing management of the following:

Complication	Pathology	Nursing Interventions
Retrolental fibroplasia		
Bronchopulmonary dysplasia		

46. As Tricia's respiratory distress decreases, monitoring her respiratory status can be done by noninvasive methods. Complete the following chart on noninvasive oxygen monitoring techniques.

Technique	Action	Nursing Responsibilities
Transcutaneous oxygen monitor (TCM)		
Pulse oximeter		

Tricia is initially maintained on intravenous fluids via umbilical catheter. When her respiratory status improves, she is placed on a half-strength premature formula via gavage feedings every 2 hours.

47. Why is gavage feeding initiated before nipple feedings?

48. List three methods of assessing proper placement of a gavage tube prior to feedings.
     a.

     b.

     c.

*49. What nursing assessments would you make to determine the following?
     a. Tricia's tolerance of gavage feedings

     b. Tricia's readiness for nipple feeding

50. What are Tricia's caloric and fluid requirements per kilogram per day?

51. Tricia's mother arrives at the special-care nursery when Tricia is 3 hours old. Describe the information and support you should give Tricia's mother.
     a. Prior to entering the nursery

     b. During her visit with Tricia

_____

*These questions are addressed at the end of Part I.

52. Why is it advised that parents have early contact with and involvement in their preterm infant's care?

53. As you talk with Tricia's mother, she expresses concern about the physical and mental development of her baby. Based on your knowledge of the growth and development of a preterm infant, how would you respond about the following areas?

   a. Physical development for the first year

   b. Mental development

   c. Emotional and social behavior

54. What criteria will be used to determine Tricia's readiness for discharge to her parents?

55. What observations would you make in assessing Tricia's parents' readiness to take Tricia home?

56. Follow-up care of preterm infants is often undertaken by the public health nurse. What information should you supply the public health nurse to facilitate Tricia's transition to home care?

At-risk infants are susceptible to temperature instability and should be placed in a regulated environment.

57. Why is it desirable to maintain an infant in a neutral thermal environment?

58. In what range should an infant's skin temperature be maintained?

If the infant's thermal environment is not maintained, cold stress can occur.

*59. What four metabolic changes and resultant problems may occur as a result of cold stress?

a.

b.

c.

d.

60. Describe the nursing interventions you would institute to prevent or minimize hypothermia/cold stress.

---

*These questions are addressed at the end of Part I.

Neonatal Jaundice

*61. List three factors that influence the rate and amount of bilirubin conjugation.

a.

b.

c.

*62. State three situations that alter the neonate's ability to conjugate bilirubin.

a.

b.

c.

63. In the following chart, compare physiologic and pathologic jaundice (hyperbilirubinemia).

Characteristic	Physiologic Jaundice	Pathologic Jaundice
Cause		
Bilirubin level in premature infant		
Bilirubin level in full-term infant		
Time of onset		

*64. What factors might influence your assessment of the neonate's developing jaundice?

*These questions are addressed at the end of Part I.

*65. **Action Sequence**—Hemolytic Disease of the Newborn

You are taking care of Alice, a 24-hour-old, 7 lb, 2 oz newborn, and her mother on the mother-baby unit. During your initial assessments and care of Alice, you notice she looks yellow. We've answered portions of this at the end of Part I.

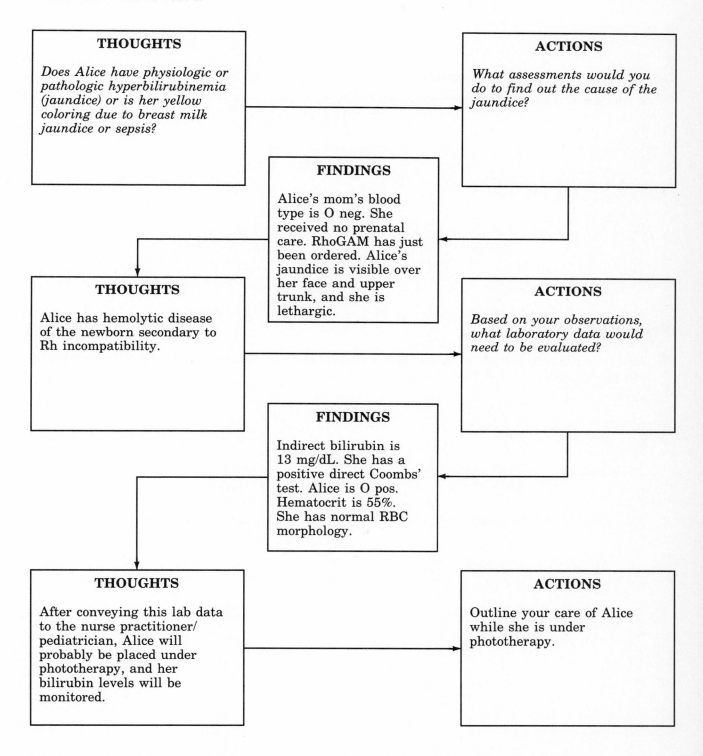

THOUGHTS

Does Alice have physiologic or pathologic hyperbilirubinemia (jaundice) or is her yellow coloring due to breast milk jaundice or sepsis?

ACTIONS

What assessments would you do to find out the cause of the jaundice?

FINDINGS

Alice's mom's blood type is O neg. She received no prenatal care. RhoGAM has just been ordered. Alice's jaundice is visible over her face and upper trunk, and she is lethargic.

THOUGHTS

Alice has hemolytic disease of the newborn secondary to Rh incompatibility.

ACTIONS

Based on your observations, what laboratory data would need to be evaluated?

FINDINGS

Indirect bilirubin is 13 mg/dL. She has a positive direct Coombs' test. Alice is O pos. Hematocrit is 55%. She has normal RBC morphology.

THOUGHTS

After conveying this lab data to the nurse practitioner/ pediatrician, Alice will probably be placed under phototherapy, and her bilirubin levels will be monitored.

ACTIONS

Outline your care of Alice while she is under phototherapy.

*These questions are addressed at the end of Part I.

66. Describe how an exchange transfusion works in the treatment of hyperbilirubinemia.

67. What are your nursing responsibilities

   a. during a neonatal exchange transfusion?

   b. following a neonatal exchange transfusion?

Neonatal Infections

68. Jane is an 8 lb baby girl whose mother had active syphilis. List eight symptoms of congenital syphilis you might expect to see during Jane's neonatal period.

   a.

   b.

   c.

   d.

   e.

   f.

   g.

   h.

*69. Describe five nursing measures you would include in your care of a baby with congenital syphilis.

a.

b.

c.

d.

e.

70. You are taking care of Andy, who is 2 days old, and note that he is increasingly lethargic and refuses to eat. He is diagnosed as having sepsis neonatorum. List four factors that increase the newborn's susceptibility to infections.

a.

b.

c.

d.

71. Identify three bacterial organisms that may cause sepsis neonatorum.

a.

b.

c.

72. List five symptoms that Andy may exhibit as manifestations of sepsis neonatorum.

    a.

    b.

    c.

    d.

    e.

*73. Identify four diagnostic tests that might be done in a septic workup.

    a.

    b.

    c.

    d.

74. What are your nursing responsibilities while caring for a septic newborn (include your rationale)?

---

*These questions are addressed at the end of Part I.

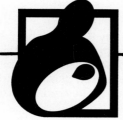

It's Your Turn

Think about a newborn with complications you have taken care of. What were the parents' responses? Describe what the experience was like for you.

_____

_____

_____

_____

_____

_____

_____

_____

_____

_____

Selected Answers

This section addresses the asterisked questions found in this chapter.

2. Baby Joey's gestational age is 36–37 weeks, which places him as being preterm, and his weight of 1500 gm places him below the tenth percentile for weight. His GA and weight classify him as a preterm SGA newborn. Based on this classification, you would want to watch Joey for the potential problems of hypothermia, respiratory distress, hypoglycemia, hypocalcemia, and polycythemia.

8. Any infant who at birth is at or below the tenth percentile on intrauterine growth charts should be suspected of being small for gestational age. If growth retardation is the result of an acute episode of placental insufficiency, observe the infant for loss of subcutaneous fat and muscle mass, a wide-eyed face, loss of vernix prior to full term, dry and desquamated skin, and the presence of a meconium-stained cord, skin, and nails in a full-term or preterm infant. By your identification of a possible SGA infant, you can be instrumental in meeting his or her immediate special needs and in reducing the possible long-term sequelae.

20. Obstetric situations that would lead you to suspect a postterm pregnancy include the following: oligohydramnios, weight loss of 3 lb or more per week in the last weeks of pregnancy, meconium-stained amniotic fluid in a full-term infant, palpation of a hard fetal head, high fetal head arrest, and prolonged labor due to uterine inertia, or CPD. Women of high parity (gravida 4 or more), primigravidas, and women whose preceding pregnancy was postterm are also more prone to go beyond term in their present pregnancy.

25. Basic preparations and equipment necessary for receiving a preterm newborn should include a method for temperature stabilization (isolette or open bed warmer) and a method for ventilatory support (oxygen, appropriate size intubation tubes and airways, and suction equipment). In addition, if appropriate for your nursery, you should provide an alternative method for supplying intravenous fluids and for monitoring blood gases (other than through the scalp veins), such as umbilical catheters. In emergency situation, a #5 feeding tube may be placed in the umbilical artery or vein. The availability of ventilatory support such as a respirator is ideal.

If you have identified the equipment necessary to provide for adequate oxygenation and temperature stabilization, you are prepared to meet the preterm infant's two most crucial initial needs.

26. The three initial assessments you should make on the arrival of a preterm newborn in the nursery area: observation of signs of respiratory distress, core temperature determination to assess whether hypothermia or cold stress will complicate this infant's course, and gestational age determination to identify other potential problems. You may have identified other areas, but these are the essential ones. Refer to your textbook if you had any difficulty identifying the initial needs of the preterm newborn.

34. If you answered "no" you were correct. Celeste is not a candidate for further resuscitation because of her vigorous crying after birth, no signs of respiratory distress, and the thin nature of the meconium-stained amniotic fluid. Vigorous resuscitation with intubation is controversial in this situation as it may do more harm to the baby.

Your most pressing nursing goal is to dry off the baby and continue assessment of respiratory function.

37. Brian probably has narcotic depression; you would give Narcan and continue ventilatory support.

39. Six signs of respiratory distress are tachypnea, inspiratory retractions, expiratory grunting, nasal flaring, cyanosis, and periods of apnea. Other signs you might look for after these six are lung rales or rhonchi, edema, and chin tug.

40. Congratulations if you scored Tricia's respiratory distress as 6. This is based on nasal flaring—1, lower chest retractions—1, xiphoid retractions—1, chest lag on inspiration—1, and expiratory grunting—2.

41. You also remembered that a lower score is desirable for this scoring system and indicates normal respiratory effort or less respiratory distress. Tricia is having significant respiratory distress: Based on her small size and early gestational age, she is using large amounts of energy in her work of breathing and will exhaust her supply of surfactant.

42. Tricia's history of preterm delivery, a low Apgar score (hypoxic insult), and a low core temperature (cold stress) are all contributing factors to her development of respiratory distress syndrome.

44. a. Nursing responsibilities during oxygen administration include ensuring that the infant's head is under the oxygen hood and that respiratory passages are not obstructed; ensuring that the tubing is connected and free of moisture buildup; seeing that ambient oxygen concentrations are being monitored by oxygen sensors; and ensuring that oxygen delivery devices are calibrated periodically.

49. a. Nursing assessments of Tricia's tolerance of gavage feedings would include observing for any degree of abdominal distention during or after the feeding; a formula residual of less than 1 mL prior to the next feeding; lack of regurgitation; and no apnea, bradycardia, cyanosis, or color changes. A program of alternate gavage and nipple feeding is recommended to decrease the possibility of fatigue during feeding.

b. Active sucking motions during and between feedings might indicate the preterm infant's readiness for nipple feeding. You would expect the preterm infant who could tolerate nipple feedings to have a weak grasp of the nipple but a strong suck and to show satiety and relief of oral tension as she feeds.

59. The metabolic effects of cold stress include competition for albumin binding sites by increased nonesterified fatty acids causing increased free circulating bilirubin; increased incidence of hypoglycemia resulting from glucose being used for thermogenesis; pulmonary vasoconstriction in response to the release of norepinephrine; and increase in oxygen consumption and metabolic acidosis as the body burns brown fat deposits. If you were successful in identifying these changes, you will also be aware that these changes may create serious life-threatening problems for an at-risk infant.

61. The three most prominent factors influencing the rate and amount of bilirubin conjugation are the following: rate of red blood cell hemolysis, degree of liver maturity, and number of available albumin binding sites. In addition, you might remember that even after the bilirubin is conjugated, it can be unconjugated via the "enterohepatic circulation" and thus cause a delay in clearing the bilirubin from the circulatory system. Also, fetal red blood cells have a shorter half-life than adult cells, which increases the rate of hemolysis.

62. Situations that alter the neonate's ability to conjugate bilirubin include the following: bacterial and viral infections; competition for albumin binding sites by drugs, particularly sulfa drugs and salicylates and nonesterified fatty acids; neonatal asphyxia, which decreases the binding affinity of bilirubin to albumin; and the many causes of increased red blood cell hemolysis, such as cephalhematoma.

64. Your assessment of developing jaundice may be affected by fluorescent nursery lights with pink tints, which mask jaundice; by blue walls and blue blankets; and by the basic pigmentation of the gumline in ethnic people of color.

65. *Thoughts:* You remember that one of the criteria for differentiating physiologic jaundice from pathologic jaundice is the time of onset. Because Alice is less than 24 hours old, it leads you to think the jaundice is pathologic in nature. Breast-feeding jaundice usually does not start until after 3 days. Sepsis is a possibility and requires further investigation.

Actions: Your nursing actions would include checking Alice's chart and her mother's chart for risk factors. As you check these charts, you find that her mother received no prenatal care, and the blood typing was done on admission. Alice's perinatal history reveals that the delivery was normal without trauma, asphyxiation, or delay of the cord clamping. Alice was scored as a term AGA newborn. You complete your physical assessment to determine the extent of the jaundice and any other significant clinical findings such as activity state and bruising.

Actions: Laboratory data that you would expect to be evaluated include indirect and direct bilirubin, blood typing, Coombs' test on Alice's blood, complete white blood count, and RBC smear.

69. In caring for a neonate with congenital syphilis, your nursing care should include the following, at least initially: isolating the infant, monitoring intake and output, swaddling the neonate for comfort, covering the neonate's hand to prevent scratching, and administering penicillin per physician orders. Support and education of the parents are also essential in fostering a positive future environment for this neonate.

73. Diagnostic tests that might be done as part of a septic workup are primarily blood, spinal, nasopharyngeal, and urine cultures. If any lesions or reddened areas are noted, cultures from these areas should also be obtained. A complete blood count, chest x ray, serology, and Gram stains of cerebrospinal fluid, urine, and umbilicus may also be required. Depending on the suspected cause of the sepsis, other tests may include x rays of various portions of the body, serum IgM level determinations, and stomach (gastric) aspirations.

Part II Self-Assessment Guide

Do you know these abbreviations?

AIDS	BPD	IDM
LGA	MAS	RDS
SGA	TNZ	UAC

Add your own abbreviations or new words you have learned:

Can you answer these questions?

The following multiple-choice questions will help you assess your knowledge of the content of this chapter. Select the best answer for each of the questions and then refer to the end of Part II to check your answers.

1. Infants of diabetic mothers are at risk for which of the following problems?
   a. Erythroblastosis fetalis
   b. Hypercalcemia
   c. Respiratory distress syndrome
   d. Seizures

2. Which of the following characteristics is indicative of a preterm newborn of 34 weeks' gestation?
   a. The scalp hair is silky and lies in silky strands.
   b. The skin is covered with lanugo except for the face.
   c. The sole creases cover the anterior two-thirds of the foot.
   d. The upper two-thirds of the pinna curves inward.

3. The nursing management of a heroin-addicted newborn experiencing withdrawal includes
   a. administration of methadone and frequent assessment of vital signs.
   b. frequent assessment of vital signs and wrapping the infant snugly in a blanket.
   c. meticulous skin and perineal care and frequent tactile stimulation.
   d. minimal tactile stimulation and the provision of loose, nonrestrictive clothing.

On April 18 at 1:45 PM, a 35-week, 1580 gm male infant named John was delivered to a 20-year-old primigravida. Questions 4 through 7 relate to this situation.

4. John is beginning to show signs of respiratory distress. Determine the priority for the following nursing interventions:

    1. Notify the physician.
    2. If cyanosis occurs, provide oxygen.
    3. Record time, symptoms, degree of symptoms, and whether oxygen relieved the symptoms of respiratory distress.
    4. Apply monitoring electrodes.
    5. Maintain a patent airway.

    a. 2, 1, 5, 4, and 3
    b. 5, 1, 2, 3, and 4
    c. 4, 2, 5, 1, and 3
    d. 5, 2, 1, 4, and 3

5. John's oxygen concentration is carefully regulated, based on his PO_2 and PCO_2 levels, because high blood levels of oxygen

    a. cause cardiac shunt closures, although the latter are not permanent.
    b. cause peripheral circulatory collapse.
    c. may cause retinal spasms, leading to the development of retrolental fibroplasia.
    d. may produce hyperbilirubinemia.

6. John has demonstrated nasal flaring, intercostal retractions, expiratory grunting, and slight cyanosis. An umbilical catheter is inserted with an intravenous infusion of 5% dextrose and water. John should also be placed in

    a. an incubator with heat control.
    b. an incubator with heat, oxygen controls, and humidity.
    c. an open bed warmer with his head slightly elevated under an oxygen hood.
    d. an open bed warmer with his head slightly elevated.

7. John's parents are very anxious when they see him with all the special equipment around him. Your best response to facilitate parent-infant interaction would be to

    a. assure them that they are fortunate to have John in a special-care nursery.
    b. explain the equipment in simple terms, have them wash their hands, and provide an opportunity for them to touch John.
    c. explain the equipment simply and discuss the viability and continued existence of John.
    d. have them wash their hands so they can touch John.

8. The neonate can contract congenital syphilis from his or her mother
    a. at birth.
    b. during the fifth month of pregnancy.
    c. during the second month of pregnancy.
    d. during the seventh month of pregnancy.

9. Which of the following signs indicate hypoglycemia in the newborn?
   a. Blotchy skin
   b. Hypertonia
   c. Jitteriness
   d. Soft, weak cry

Mrs Carla Steffens, at 38 weeks' gestation, is concerned that her baby may be born with hemolytic anemia of the newborn. Questions 10 through 13 relate to this situation.

10. You would respond to Carla's concern based on your knowledge that hemolytic disease of the neonate may be produced by the union of
    a. Rh negative mother with Rh negative father.
    b. Rh negative mother with Rh positive father.
    c. Rh positive mother with Rh negative father.
    d. type O mother with type O father.

11. A positive direct Coombs' test done on the cord blood of Carla's baby indicates the presence of
    a. antibodies coating the baby's red blood cells.
    b. antigens coating the mother's red blood cells.
    c. fetal red blood cells in the maternal serum.
    d. maternal red blood cells in the fetal circulation.

12. Baby boy Steffens develops jaundice, and intravenous albumin is ordered. Albumin helps to reduce his blood bilirubin level because
    a. albumin combined with enzymes couples with the bilirubin, which can then be excreted.
    b. albumin functions as a catalyst in converting bilirubin to biliverdin, which is then excreted.
    c. bilirubin binds to albumin and is transported to the liver for excretion.
    d. bilirubin production is prevented by maintaining high levels of blood albumin.

13. Nursing interventions for baby boy Steffens should include
    a. maintaining NPO status to prevent nausea and vomiting.
    b. observation for hypothermia resulting from phototherapy.
    c. observation for low-pitched cry, which may indicate kernicterus.
    d. shielding infant's eyes during phototherapy.

Answers

1. c	2. b	3. b	4. d	5. c	6. b	7. b
8. b	9. c	10. b	11. a	12. c	13. d	

Nursing Assessment and Care of the Postpartal Family

14

Introduction

The puerperium is a time of major physiologic and psychologic adaptations as the body completes its adjustment following childbirth. This chapter begins with questions on theoretical data about common physiologic and psychologic changes. The remainder of the chapter emphasizes clinical application of the nursing process in providing care for the postpartal family and corresponds to Chapters 33, 34, and 35 in *Maternal-Newborn Nursing: A Family-Centered Approach,* 4th ed.

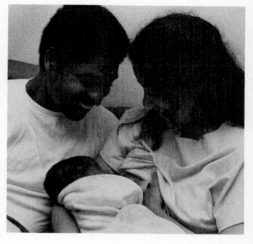

Part I Concepts, Critical Thinking, and Clinical Applications

1. Complete the following chart:

Physiologic Feature	Expected Changes	Physiologic Rationale
Uterus	Size	
	Muscle tone	
	Placental site	
	Lochia (types)	
	Lochia odor	
	Amount	

Continued

Physiologic Feature	Expected Changes	Physiologic Rationale
Cervix		
Vagina		
Perineum		
Abdomen		
Breasts		
Gastrointestinal tract		
Urinary tract		
Kidneys		
Ureters		
Bladder		
Urinary output		
Vital signs		
Blood values		
Weight changes		

2. Explain the physiologic mechanisms that cause each of the following:
   a. Postpartal chill

   b. Postpartal diaphoresis

   c. Afterpains

3. During the postpartal period, what psychologic adaptations does a new mother face?

4. Describe "postpartum blues."

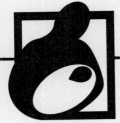

It's Your Turn

Think about a woman you have cared for postpartally or someone you have visited soon after the birth of a child (perhaps this may apply to you). What were her emotions like? Did she share her feelings with you? Did she show any signs of the postpartum blues?

_____

_____

_____

_____

_____

_____

_____

_____

_____

_____

_____

_____

_____

_____

_____

_____

_____

_____

_____

5. Name and briefly describe the four stages of maternal role attainment:

    a.

    b.

    c.

    d.

Clinical Applications

*6. Identify nine areas that should be examined during the initial postpartal *physical* assessment and then at least daily until the woman is discharged. (Do not include psychologic assessment or information needs.)

    a.

    b.

    c.

    d.

    e.

    f.

    g.

    h.

    i.

---

*These questions are addressed at the end of Part I.

7. Describe three observations you should make in assessing the breasts of a woman postpartally. Include your rationale for each.

    a.

    b.

    c.

As part of your postpartum assessment, you palpate your client's abdomen.

8. Define *diastasis rectus abdominis*. How does it occur, and how is it measured?

9. Why is it necessary to assess the fundus following childbirth?

    a. What is the significance of a well-contracted uterus?

    b. Why is the client asked to empty her bladder before you assess her fundus?

    c. Describe the correct procedure for evaluating descent of the fundus.

    d. How is fundal height recorded (according to your agency's policy)?

10. It is the second postpartal day for Megan Davenport, a 21-year-old primipara. Yesterday her fundus was one fingerbreadth below the umbilicus. Where would you expect it to be today?

11. What characteristics should be noted in assessing Megan's lochia?

12. How do you record your findings about the lochia (according to your agency's policy)?

13. When getting up to go to the bathroom after awakening on her second postpartal day, Megan becomes alarmed when she notices a sudden increase in her lochia. You check her fundus, and it is firm. How might you explain this occurrence?

14. In preparation for assessing Megan's perineum, you would have her assume the
_____ position.

15. List and explain the significance of the components of the REEDA scale in evaluating the condition of the episiotomy, if one is present.

Component	Significance
R _____	
E _____	
E _____	
D _____	
A _____	

16. What observations about the condition of the client's anal area should be made during the assessment of the perineum?

17. What information regarding the client's urinary elimination should you elicit during your physical assessment?

18. What information about your client's intestinal elimination should you elicit during your physical assessment?

19. Discuss the teaching implications of your findings on intestinal elimination.

20. Why is it important to include an evaluation of your client's lower extremities as part of your postpartal assessment?

21. How is Homan's sign elicited?

The following action sequence is designed to help you think through basic clinical problems. We've answered portions of it at the end of Part I.

*22. **Action Sequence**
Margo Jessup gave birth at 0200. At 0830 you are completing her morning postpartum assessment. You find her fundus at one fingerbreadth above the umbilicus and displaced to the right side.

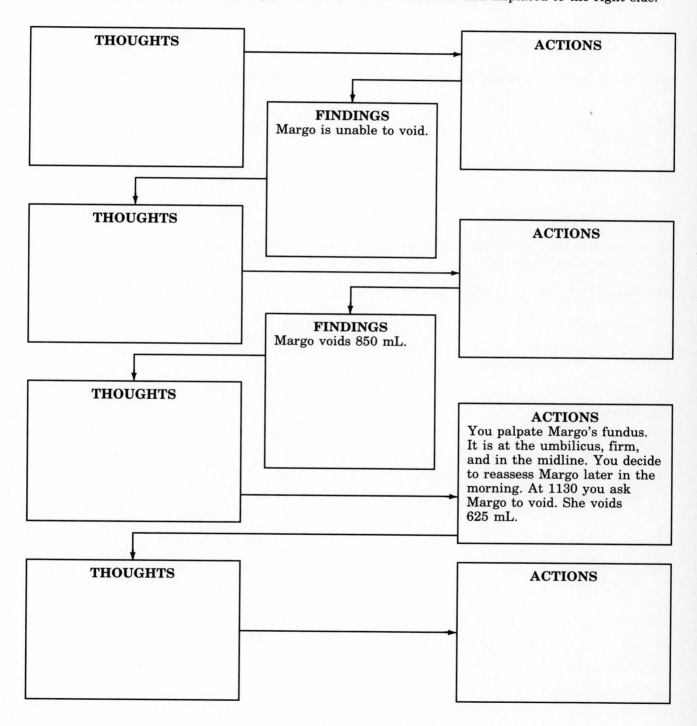

THOUGHTS

ACTIONS

FINDINGS
Margo is unable to void.

THOUGHTS

ACTIONS

FINDINGS
Margo voids 850 mL.

THOUGHTS

ACTIONS
You palpate Margo's fundus. It is at the umbilicus, firm, and in the midline. You decide to reassess Margo later in the morning. At 1130 you ask Margo to void. She voids 625 mL.

THOUGHTS

ACTIONS

*These questions are addressed at the end of Part I.

23. What assessments are important in evaluating your client's nutritional status?

24. Discuss factors you should consider in completing a psychologic assessment postpartally.

25. For each of the discomforts listed below, identify suitable comfort measures that can be instituted and the rationale for each.

Discomfort	Comfort Measures	Rationale
Episiotomy		
Hemorrhoids		
Afterpains		
Immobility		
Diaphoresis		

26. Suppression of lactation in nonnursing mothers may be done by drug therapy or by mechanical methods. Compare these approaches.

   a. Drug therapy

   b. Mechanical methods

27. You are assisting Edna Lewis to the bathroom for the first time following childbirth.

   a. What nursing assessments should you make before Edna gets up?

   b. What teaching regarding perineal hygiene should you initiate at this time?

   c. Edna decides to remain in the bathroom and take a shower after she voids. What precautions should you take to ensure her safety?

28. During the postpartal period, you may be asked to administer several of the drugs listed in the chart on the next page. For each drug, state the action/use, dose, side effects/untoward effects, and nursing considerations. Space has also been provided for you to add drugs commonly used in your agency.

Drug**	Action/Use	Dose	Excretion in Breast Milk	Side Effects/ Untoward Effects	Nursing Considerations
Methergine					
Parlodel					
Dialose					
Surfak					
Annusol HC suppository					
Ferrous sulfate					
Empirin #3					
Percodan					
RhoGAM					
Rubella vaccine					

**This list is a sample. You are encouraged to substitute any drugs that are commonly used on your unit.

29. Identify factors that influence a new mother's psychologic adjustment to childbirth and her newborn.

30. How can a nurse provide emotional support during this time?

31. You are caring for a woman who gave birth to a healthy infant the previous day. When you enter her room, she is crying. She states, "I don't know what's wrong with me. I feel as let down as if it were the day after Christmas, and I can't seem to stop crying. What's going on? Do you know why I'm acting like this?" How would you respond?

32. Freda and Earl Marshall express concern about the possible reaction of their 3-year-old son, Roy, to the birth of their daughter. Briefly describe some actions they might take to help Roy more easily adjust to the arrival of his sister.

33. Freda asks you about postpartal exercises. Develop an appropriate exercise plan and specify on which postpartal day each exercise may begin.

34. Freda asks when she and her husband can resume sexual activity. How would you respond?

35. Your instructor asks you to prepare a brief class presentation comparing rooming-in and mother-baby units. Identify their similarities and differences. What are the advantages and disadvantages for the new mother who chooses one of these approaches rather than the more traditional approach in which the newborn remains in the nursery and is brought to the mother for feeding?

*36. In many postpartal units the focus of care and attention is the mother and her newborn. Describe how you would incorporate the father or support person into your focus of care.

---

*These questions are addressed at the end of Part I.

*37. In addition to her name, age, and social history, what information would you consider essential to have as part of your data base in planning care for a woman postpartally?

38. Carla Roberts, age 29, gravida 3 para 2, gave birth to an 8 lb, 7 oz boy at 3:15 AM. Her labor lasted 18 hours, and the baby was born by low forceps. She received no medication during labor but did have a pudendal block for birth. She had a midline episiotomy and a third-degree extension. She also has two large hemorrhoids. The baby had an Apgar score of 7 at 1 minute and 9 at 5 minutes. He is apparently healthy, although he has a large bruise on each temple from the forceps and pronounced molding of his head. The labor nurse reported that Harry Roberts, Carla's husband, was present at the birth and expressed great pleasure at the birth of his third son. Carla was openly disappointed that the newborn was not the girl she had so greatly desired.

It is now 8 AM. Carla has just finished breakfast, and you are assigned as her nurse today. Carla has voided twice since birth: 700 mL and 550 mL. Her fundus has remained firm and is at the umbilicus. Her lochia is rubra and moderate. Her vital signs are normal, and she is a breast-feeding mother. Her orders include a shower; a sitz bath TID; Dermaplast spray p.r.n.; up ad lib.; Tylenol #3 q.4h p.r.n.; a regular diet; fluids; a straight catheter × 1 p.r.n. for marked distention; and Surfak 1 capsule b.i.d.

*a. What do you consider the two highest priorities in planning Carla's physical care?

b. Develop a plan of care for the morning based on your assessment of Carla's condition. Include the appropriate rationale.
Patient care goals:

*These questions are addressed at the end of Part I.

Nursing Diagnosis and Supporting Data	Nursing Interventions	Rationale

Evaluation:

*c. You know that disappointment over the sex of an infant may produce problems in maternal-infant bonding. Identify two ways in which you can assess Carla for potential attachment problems.

d. In observing Carla with her new son, what behavior might she exhibit that would indicate healthy maternal-infant attachment?

e. What behaviors might Carla exhibit that would suggest possible failure to bond well?

*These questions are addressed at the end of Part I.

39. How does postpartum assessment and care differ for the woman who gives birth by cesarean?

40. Patient-controlled analgesia (PCA) is becoming increasingly popular.

    a. Describe how it is used.

    b. How is the client on PCA protected from overdose?

41. Discuss approaches a nurse can use to promote maternal-infant attachment for the cesarean birth mother.

42. Describe some of the special nursing needs of the adolescent mother postpartally.

43. How can the postpartum nurse provide support and assistance to a woman who is relinquishing her infant?

44. Vicky and Larry Darnell are preparing to take their first child, Lori, home today. Vicky is planning to bottle-feed Lori. Vicky had an uncomplicated labor and birth but has a small midline episiotomy that has caused some discomfort. You are assigned to Mrs Darnell today and are responsible for discharge teaching. Describe what information you will include in your discharge teaching for the following areas:

   a. Care of the episiotomy

   b. Rest

   c. Activity and exercises

   d. Resumption of sexual activity and birth control methods

   e. Symptoms in the mother that should be reported

   f. Support systems

   g. Baby care

   h. Symptoms in the baby that should be reported

   i. Infant safety (crib, car seat)

   j. Follow-up medical care for both mother and infant

   k. Community resources

45. Naomi Carlson gave birth her first child in the birthing room 8 hours ago. Now she is preparing for discharge.

    a. Describe how you will explain the reasons for and importance of returning to the hospital for a test for phenylketonuria and other metabolic disorders.

    *b. As part of your follow-up experience, you will be accompanying a registered nurse on a visit to Naomi's home tomorrow. List the assessments you should make on your home visit.

Mother	Newborn	Educational Needs

Selected Answers

This section addresses the asterisked questions found in this chapter.

6. The following essential areas need to be included in your daily physical assessment of the postpartal client:

    a. Vital signs
    b. Breasts, including nipples
    c. Fundus and abdomen
    d. Lochia
    e. Perineum (including the anus)
    f. Elimination
    g. Lower extremities
    h. Nutritional status
    i. Activity level

    If you listed most of these, you are well on your way to providing good nursing care for your clients. If you missed three or more, you need to refer back to the postpartum section in your textbook. Other areas that may be considered are the discomfort level and sleep patterns.

---

*These questions are addressed at the end of Part I.

22.   *Thoughts:* You suspect that Ms Jessup's bladder is distended. You know that because the uterine ligaments are still stretched, a distended bladder can easily displace the uterus and cause it to appear higher in the abdomen. It may also keep the uterus from remaining firmly contracted.

Actions: You assist Ms Jessup to the bathroom so she can attempt to void. You place a "Johnny cap" under the seat of the commode so you can measure her output. You show her where the call light is, and you leave her in privacy to attempt to void.

Thoughts: You know that a distended bladder is common postpartally. You also know that pressure and trauma can reduce bladder sensitivity and tone. However, if Ms Jessup is not able to void, it may be necessary to catheterize her. You hope to avoid catheterization because of the associated risk of infection.

Actions: You employ nursing measures to assist Ms Jessup. You pour a measured amount of warm water slowly over her perineum while her wrist is resting in warm water. You also create a verbal picture of flowing water for her. You encourage her to use her other hand to massage her bladder.

Thoughts: You are pleased that Ms Jessup has been able to void successfully. You decide to reassess her uterus to be certain it is now firm.

Thoughts: The fact that Ms Jessup has been able to void two large amounts suggests that her bladder tone is adequate.

Actions: You tell Ms Jessup that you think she is doing well. You point out that incomplete emptying of the bladder can lead to a boggy uterus and may also contribute to the development of a bladder infection. You ask her to monitor her next two or three voidings and report to the nurse if she feels that she is not emptying her bladder fully or if she begins voiding in small amounts.

Nice job! You made accurate assessments and employed nursing actions effectively. You also treated Ms Jessup like a responsible adult by explaining the situation and involving her in assuming responsibility for her own care.

36.   The father or support person can be included more readily by
      a.   encouraging him or her to visit whenever possible during the day or evening and to participate in infant care.
      b.   encouraging him or her to come in for infant feeding.
      c.   including him or her in parenting classes in the postpartal unit.
      d.   being supportive of his or her efforts.
      e.   providing time for any question.
      f.   including him or her in all teaching.
      These are just a few possibilities. You may have thought of others.

37.   You should include information about her obstetric history, including the following:
      a.   Number of pregnancies, births, and abortions
      b.   Significant prenatal problems and conditions
      c.   Date and time of birth
      d.   Medications given (anesthesia and analgesics)
      e.   Course of labor and birth (for example, time of rupture of membranes; use of forceps, episiotomy, prolonged second stage)
      f.   Sex, Apgar score, and present condition of the infant, along with pertinent recovery room data
      g.   Available support systems. (In many agencies the mother's marital status has little relevance. The focus is on the support she has available to her.)

h. Any existing problems or complaints (including allergies to food or drugs)

i. Method of feeding the infant

j. Teaching needs

If you included most of this information, you are on the right track. If you included the physical aspects but neglected the support and teaching areas, you may find it helpful to review material related to psychologic adjustments and teaching needs during the early postpartal period.

38. a. High on your list of priorities in planning Carla's physical care should be rest and comfort. With an 18-hour labor, you know she has been up all night and most of the preceding day. Her third-degree extension and hemorrhoids make comfort important, and meeting this need will enable her to rest more easily.

Because this is probably her first shower, safety is a fairly high priority, as it is with most women following birth.

If you listed bladder or intestinal elimination as a high priority, you may wish to review your textbook.

It is always pertinent to assess a postpartal woman for hemorrhage, but since her fundus has remained firm, it would not be your highest priority.

c. You can assess Carla's attitude toward her child by unobtrusively observing her with her infant and by discussing the subject with her in an open, nonjudgmental way. Although her history suggests a possible bonding problem, it is not appropriate to jump to conclusions without further data. Frequently parents will express initial disappointment about a child's sex or behavior and then bond beautifully later.

45. b. The postpartal home visit should include assessment of the following:

Mother	Newborn	Educational Needs
Vital signs	Vital signs	Self-care
Breasts	Skin color and rashes	Baby care
Fundus	Umbilical cord	
Lochia	Feedings	
Episiotomy	Voiding and stooling pattern	
Bladder	Sleep pattern	
Bowels	Alertness	
Rest and nutrition		
Mother-infant interaction		
Support systems		

Congratulations if you included all (or most) of these items. If you had trouble with this question, you need to refer to the postpartal assessment guide in your textbook.

Part II Self-Assessment Guide

The following multiple-choice questions will help you assess your knowledge of the content of this chapter. Select the best answer for each of the questions and then refer to the end of Part II to check your answers.

Questions 1–4 pertain to the following situation. Joyce Palmer, a 24-year-old gravida 1 para 1, gave birth to Bryan, an 8-lb full-term infant. She is nursing her infant. She had a midline episiotomy. It is her first postpartal day. As part of your daily postpartal care, you assess each of the following systems for signs that they are functioning normally.

1. The fundus should be
    a. at the level of the symphysis pubis.
    b. at the level of the umbilicus.
    c. midway between the umbilicus and symphysis pubis.
    d. two fingerbreadths below the umbilicus.

2. The lochia should have a
    a. characteristic foul odor and be blood mixed with a small amount of mucus.
    b. characteristic foul odor and be dark brown with occasional red bleeding.
    c. fleshy odor and be clear-colored and moderate in amount.
    d. fleshy odor with blood and a small amount of mucus mixed in.

3. The perineum should be
    a. edematous, painful to pressure, and displaying a clear discharge.
    b. edematous, painful to pressure, and perhaps displaying hemorrhoids.
    c. intensely painful in the episiotomy area and displaying clear drainage.
    d. displaying clear drainage and perhaps hemorrhoids.

4. The breasts should be
    a. full and secreting colostrum.
    b. engorged and secreting colostrum.
    c. soft and secreting milk.
    d. engorged and not secreting any fluid.

5. Uterine involution occurs as a result of
    a. a decrease in the number of myometrial cells.
    b. necrosis of the hypertrophic myometrial cells.
    c. autolysis of protein material within the uterine wall.
    d. necrotic degeneration of the placental site.

6. Mrs Chang is a gravida 2 para 2. While assessing her fundus 12 hours after birth, you find that it is enlarged and boggy. What would be your first nursing intervention?
    a. Take her vital signs.
    b. Check the consistency of her fundus at 15-minute intervals.
    c. Administer an oxytocic drug.
    d. Massage the uterus firmly with one hand while supporting it with the other hand.

7. Which of the following instructions should be given to a postpartal mother about perineal care?
   a. Cleansing the area should be a sterile procedure.
   b. The area should be cleansed from front to back.
   c. A sterilized perineal pad should be applied to the perineum.
   d. An antiseptic should be used to cleanse the perineum to prevent inflammation.

8. Difficulty in voiding after childbirth may be due to which of the following factors?
   a. Decreased sensitivity of the bladder
   b. Lack of food and fluid intake during labor
   c. Relaxation of the abdominal wall
   d. All of the above

9. During the day or so following childbirth, as the mother works to adjust psychologically to her experience, she tends to be most concerned about
   a. details of her birth and herself.
   b. planning for her discharge.
   c. her new infant's needs and care.
   d. postpartal exercises for herself.

Answers

1. b   2. d   3. b   4. a   5. c   6. d   7. b   8. d   9. a

The Postpartal Family at Risk

15

Introduction

The postpartal period is regarded by some as rather anticlimactic. The great drama of labor and birth is completed, and there seems to be little else to do. In reality, this is far from true. After even the most uneventful birth, nursing assessments of mother and baby are essential. The emotional support and teaching a postpartal nurse provides cannot be overemphasized, nor can the nurse's responsibility to carefully monitor the mother's physical status. Complications do sometimes develop during the postpartal period, but their severity may often be ameliorated by early detection and intervention.

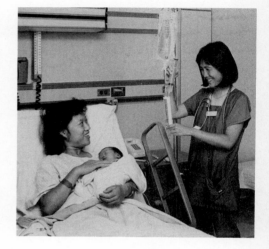

This chapter is designed to explore the complications that may arise during the postpartal period. It begins with hemorrhage, the major risk for the childbearing mother. It then goes on to consider other potential complications and ends with disorders of bonding. This chapter corresponds to Chapter 36 in *Maternal-Newborn Nursing: A Family-Centered Approach,* 4th ed.

Part I Concepts, Critical Thinking, and Clinical Applications

Postpartum Hemorrhage

1. Postpartum hemorrhage may be classified as early or late. Describe the time of onset and primary cause(s) of each.

   a. Early

   b. Late

2. List five contributing factors that would predispose a mother to postpartum hemorrhage.

   a.

   b.

   c.

   d.

   e.

Joan Burke, a 33-year-old gravida 3 para 3, is recovering following the birth of twin boys. Her labor lasted 2 1/2 hours.

*3. Identify two factors that predispose Joan to early postpartum hemorrhage.

   a.

   b.

4. During your assessment of Joan, what three findings would indicate possible postpartum hemorrhage?

   a.

   b.

   c.

*5. Your nursing assessment indicates that Joan is having an early postpartum hemorrhage. Formulate an appropriate nursing diagnosis.

*6. What do you consider the two highest priorities in planning your care of Joan?

7. What nursing interventions should be initiated for Joan as she demonstrates signs of postpartum hemorrhage?

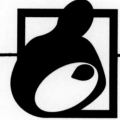

It's Your Turn

Have you provided care for a woman experiencing bleeding in the immediate postpartum period? What concerns did she express? Describe the experience for you.

_____

_____

_____

_____

_____

_____

_____

_____

_____

_____

_____

Subinvolution

Mrs Gloria Brown, a breast-feeding mother, gave birth to a 8 lb 11 1/2 oz baby boy, Vincent, vaginally after Pitocin augmentation. She has been home for 2 weeks and calls the office. She tells the Ob/Gyn nurse-practitioner that she is concerned because her flow has increased and is red but not foul smelling.

*8. Identify nursing assessments that might lead you to suspect subinvolution.

*9. After assessing Mrs Brown's complaints, formulate an appropriate nursing diagnosis.

10. Based on your nursing diagnosis, identify three nursing interventions to meet Mrs Brown's needs.

---

*These questions are addressed at the end of Part I.

*11. **Action Sequence**

The following action sequence is designed to help you think through basic clinical problems. We have answered portions of it at the end of Part I.

You are taking care of Mrs Carrie Spencer, age 24, G1 P1, on the mother-baby unit. She is 8 hours postbirth of an 8 lb 2 oz baby girl. As you are carrying out her postpartal assessments, she complains of tenderness and pain in her perineal area. She says, "My stitches hurt; it feels as if they are tearing apart."

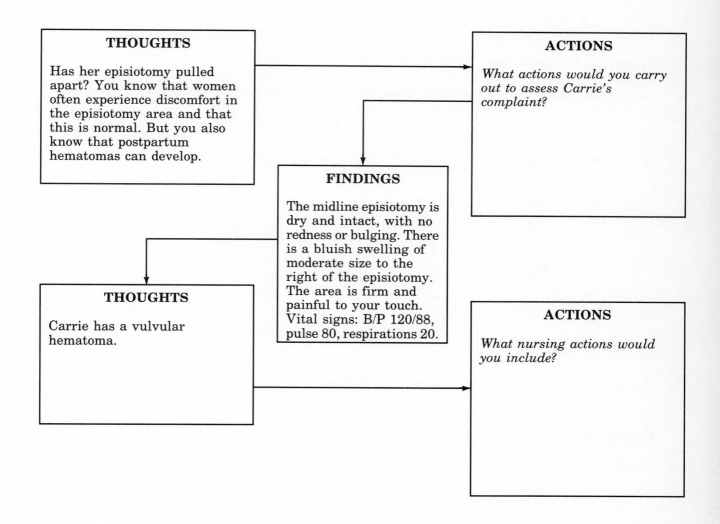

THOUGHTS

Has her episiotomy pulled apart? You know that women often experience discomfort in the episiotomy area and that this is normal. But you also know that postpartum hematomas can develop.

ACTIONS

What actions would you carry out to assess Carrie's complaint?

FINDINGS

The midline episiotomy is dry and intact, with no redness or bulging. There is a bluish swelling of moderate size to the right of the episiotomy. The area is firm and painful to your touch. Vital signs: B/P 120/88, pulse 80, respirations 20.

THOUGHTS

Carrie has a vulvular hematoma.

ACTIONS

What nursing actions would you include?

---

*These questions are addressed at the end of Part I.

12. Describe the anticipated treatment of Carrie's problem.

Puerperal Infections

13. Identify the physiologic reasons why a woman during labor and birth has an increased susceptibility to infection.

    a.

    b.

    c.

    d.

14. Complete the following chart on puerperal infection:

Component	Localized Infection (Episiotomy and/ or Laceration)	Endometritis	Parametritis
Tissues involved			
Clinical manifestations			
Interventions			
Complications			

*15. Identify evaluative outcome criteria findings that indicate your interventions/treatments of puerperal infection have been effective.

Thromboembolic Disease

16. Match the following descriptive statements with the correct thromboembolic disease.

a. Superficial thrombophlebitis   _____ Clotting process involving the saphenous vein system

b. Deep vein thrombosis   _____ More frequently seen in women with history of thrombosis

c. Pulmonary embolism   _____ Usually appears about third or fourth postpartal day

     _____ Sudden onset of sweating, pallor, dyspnea, and chest pain

     _____ Prompt intervention with heparin, oxygen, and lidocaine as needed

     _____ Edema of ankle and leg; low-grade fever and positive Homan's sign

     _____ Treatment primarily involves intravenous heparin and bed rest

     _____ Management principally involves leg elevation, moist packs, bedrest, and elastic stockings

17. Discuss the physiologic changes of pregnancy that increase a woman's susceptibility to blood clot formation during the postpartal period.

18. List two diagnostic tests used to identify superficial thrombophlebitis.

a.

b.

---

*These questions are addressed at the end of Part I.

19. Identify three interventions useful in preventing the development of thrombophlebitis during the postpartal period.

    a.

    b.

    c.

20. Describe the appropriate interventions for a mother with deep vein thrombosis.

21. What medication would you expect a woman with deep vein thrombosis to receive initially?

22. Identify three signs of anticoagulant overdose.

    a.

    b.

    c.

23. The antagonist of heparin is _____ .

24. What education for self-care should be given to a woman receiving Warfarin (Coumadin)?

*25. The following situation has been included to challenge your critical thinking. Read the situation and then answer the question "yes" or "no."

Joan McGuire, age 34, Gr 3 P 3, gave birth to twin boys vaginally with regional anesthesia 12 hours ago and you are now responsible for her care. She complains of cramping when the uterus attempts to contract. Your assessment reveals a uterus one fingerbreadth above the umbilicus and displaced to the right and increased vaginal bleeding.

Is Mrs McGuire a candidate for bladder distention?

⇓   ⇓

Yes (Why? _____)   No (Why not? _____)
Identify the therapy you would expect to   Identify your most pressing nursing goal.
be initiated.

Puerperal Cystitis

26. List three factors that predispose the postpartal woman to the development of cystitis.

a.

b.

c.

27. Identify appropriate interventions in the treatment of the postpartal woman with cystitis.

---

*These questions are addressed at the end of Part I.

Mastitis

One week after her discharge, Alice Enriquez, a 23-year-old gravida 1 para 1 breast-feeding mother, develops mastitis.

28. List two factors that contribute to the development of mastitis.

   a.

   b.

29. Identify four clinical manifestations of mastitis that Alice may exhibit.

   a.

   b.

   c.

   d.

Two nursing diagnoses that may apply to Alice are "Acute pain related to inflammation and swelling of breast tissue" and "Knowledge deficit related to appropriate breast-feeding techniques."

30. Based on these possible nursing diagnoses, describe the interventions Alice or you may institute.

31. Compare the various opinions about continuing breast-feeding during an episode of mastitis.

32. In evaluating the nursing diagnosis "Knowledge deficit related to appropriate breast-feeding techniques," identify the evaluative outcome criteria that would indicate that Alice's knowledge about breast-feeding during mastitis has changed.

It is the third postpartal day for Bonnie Sumpter, an 18-year-old primipara. She is single and is keeping her baby. In team conference her nurse expresses concern that she is not bonding appropriately with her infant.

33. Identify four behaviors that might indicate inadequate maternal bonding.

   a.

   b.

   c.

   d.

34. Discuss ways in which the nurse can assist Bonnie in bonding with her infant.

Selected Answers

This section addresses the asterisked questions found in this chapter.

3. Joan is predisposed to early postpartum hemorrhage because of overdistention of the uterus, which is present with a full-term multiple pregnancy, and because of her precipitous labor.

5. The nursing diagnosis you developed, "Potential fluid volume deficit related to blood loss," is an important one. Joan is at risk for bleeding secondary to uterine atony. This nursing diagnosis would alert you to intervene if she demonstrates signs of early postpartal bleeding. Another possible nursing diagnosis is "Anxiety related to excessive bleeding."

6. Early identification of and management of uterine relaxation/atony and blood loss are high priorities. Another high priority is assisting Joan and her husband to deal with the anxiety over her bleeding.

8. Two key nursing assessments that would lead you to suspect subinvolution are failure of the uterus to decrease in size at the expected rate and prolongation of lochia rubra or return of lochia rubra after the first several days of the postpartal period. Breast-feeding assists in involution, as you know, but you should not rule out the possibility of subinvolution in breast-feeding mothers if these signs exist.

9. Nursing diagnoses involved in subinvolution might include "Knowledge deficit related to lack of understanding of signs of subinvolution" and "Fatigue related to blood loss."

11. *Actions:* As you assess Carrie's episiotomy for redness, swelling, warmth, and intactness, you would also visualize and palpate her total perineal area to assess for hematoma development.

Actions: Your nursing actions to improve comfort would include application of covered ice packs to decrease the swelling and discomfort. You may also use sitz baths to aid in fluid absorption and give analgesics as ordered and needed. You may also encourage her to void to avoid the need for catheterization. Careful observation and palpation of this site are essential so that you can assess any extension or enlargement of the hematoma. Frequent monitoring of vital signs q. 15 min will enable you to assess any blood loss and the possible development of shock. You would also notify her physician of any increase in the size of the hematoma or changes in vital signs. Discomfort experienced by women after delivery is often overlooked. By your thought processes and nursing actions, you have done much to alleviate her discomfort.

15. Evaluative outcome criteria would include:
    a. Exhibits signs of wound healing, such as decreased drainage, swelling, or redness of tissues.
    b. Has a normal temperature.
    c. Demonstrates increased tolerance for ambulation.
    d. Woman understands treatment regimen, self-care, preventive measures, and implications for the care of her newborn.

    Your evaluative outcome criteria may differ from these but should address some of these aspects.

25. Joan McGuire is at risk for overdistention of her bladder. Her risk factors included regional anesthesia and birth of twins (overdistention of the uterus). In addition, your physical findings which would support your response of "yes" are; the uterus is above the umbilicus and displaced to the right (by the distended bladder) and an increase in vaginal bleeding because the uterus cannot contract adequately.

    Initial therapy is directed toward assisting her to empty her bladder for example, pouring warm water over the perineum or having her void in the sitz bath, providing pain medication as needed prior to her attempt to void, and applying ice packs to the perineum immediately postpartum to minimize edema, which can interfere with voiding. If these measures don't assist Joan to void then catheterization may be done.

Part II Self-Assessment Guide

Do you know this abbreviation?

REEDA

Add your own abbreviations or new words you have learned:

Can you answer these questions?

The following multiple-choice questions will help you assess your knowledge of the content of this chapter. Select the best answer for each of the questions and then refer to the end of Part II to check your answers.

1. A neighbor who had a cesarean birth 10 days ago calls to ask your advice. She tells you that she has lochia rubra and is still using eight maternity pads a day. You would suspect which of the following?
   a. Endometritis
   b. Nothing, because this is normal course for a cesarean birth
   c. Parametritis
   d. Subinvolution

2. Maggie Applegate, Gr 3 P 2, had a healthy 3850 gm boy following a lengthy labor and vaginal birth with low forceps. On the second postpartum day, Maggie complains that she is very uncomfortable sitting on the side of the bed and has a "full feeling down there." You would suspect which of the following?

    a. Cystitis
    b. Postpartum hemorrhage
    c. Postpartum infection
    d. Vulvar hematoma

3. The clinical manifestations of a localized infection of the episiotomy would include

    a. approximation of skin edges of the episiotomy.
    b. patient complaint of severe discomfort in the perineum and an oral temperature of 99.8 °F (37.7 °C).
    c. reddened, bruised tissue.
    d. reddened, edematous tissue with yellowish discharge.

Marie Walker has recently given birth and states that she has a history of thrombophlebitis. Questions 4 through 8 are related to Marie's condition.

4. Which of the following nursing measures will be most important for Marie in light of her history?

    a. Assess vital signs frequently.
    b. Encourage early ambulation.
    c. Encourage Marie to rest in bed with the knee gatch up.
    d. Maintain bed rest.

5. Marie has developed thrombophlebitis and is receiving heparin intravenously. It will be important to watch her for signs of overdose, which include

    a. dysuria.
    b. epistaxis, hematuria, and dysuria.
    c. hematuria, ecchymosis, and epistaxis.
    d. hematuria, ecchymosis, and vertigo.

6. You know that a drug used to combat problems related to overdoses of heparin is

    a. calcium gluconate.
    b. calcium sulfate.
    c. protamine sulfate.
    d. protamine zinc.

7. As you talk with Marie, she suddenly complains of dyspnea and chest pain. Marie has developed

    a. a drug reaction to heparin.
    b. an inflammatory reaction.
    c. another thrombophlebitis.
    d. pulmonary embolism.

8. A positive Homan's sign is indicated by a complaint of pain in

    a. the foot when the patient stands.
    b. the leg when the foot is dorsiflexed while the knee is held flat.
    c. the leg when the knee is flexed and the foot is extended.
    d. the leg when the knee is held flat and the foot is rotated.

9. Which of the following assessments would indicate an overdistended bladder?

    a. A lower pelvic mass
    b. Complaints of discomfort while voiding
    c. Positive Homan's sign
    d. Voiding measured at 200 cc

10. Naomi Brookens, a breast-feeding mother, develops mastitis. The clinical manifestations of mastitis include

    a. a hard, warm nodular area in the outer quadrant of the breast.
    b. cessation of lactation.
    c. marked engorgement and pain.
    d. marked engorgement, high temperature, chills, and pain.

Answers

1. d	2. d	3. d	4. b	5. c
6. c	7. d	8. b	9. a	10. a